OUR STORIES TO TELL

OUR STORIES TO TELL

Edited by
Hannah Fields

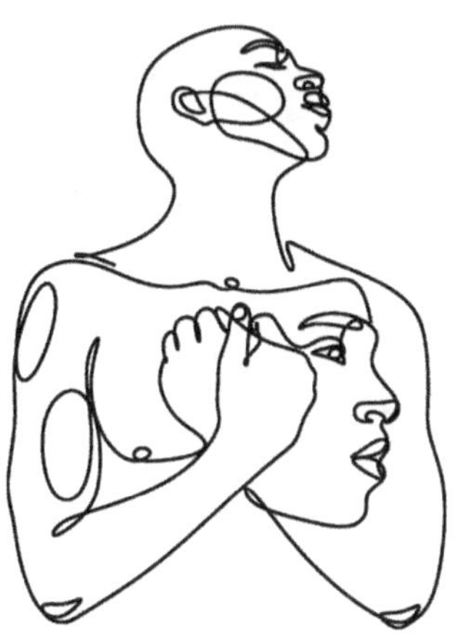

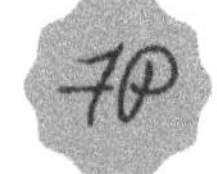

FOLKWAYS PRESS, LLC

Texas, USA
www.folkwayspress.com

Our Stories to Tell first published in 2022

ISBN: 978-1-7362701-1-0

CONTENTS

OUR STORIES TO TELL

INTRODUCTION

Not a Whisper, but a Roar

For as long as I can remember, mental health has always carried some sort of taboo air about it – as if it were a dirty word that would make others blush or turn in disgust at just the mention of it. Because of this, there are so many people who don't get the help they need, usually out of fear of how they will be perceived by those closest to them, or society in general. This isn't surprising when much of the media we consume constantly frames mental-ill health in a negative light – whether that be by casting mentally ill characters as villains or by framing mental illness as the sole cause of violent acts we see reported on the nightly news. With such negative connotations being put on full volume, all others become a whisper – that being one of the many reasons I was inspired to put this anthology together. I don't want to be a whisper, I want to be a voice rising above the noise, and I want others to feel brave in that same way when speaking up about mental health.

I first felt something was "off" within myself when I was thirteen or fourteen years old. There's always talk of "teen angst" or "raging hormones," but it was something so much more than that. Thinking back, I remember not having any motivation for the things I once loved, like participating in band and sports or spending time with friends

– yet went through the motions anyway. In addition, I often had thoughts of wanting to end my life, thinking that was probably the only option I had for ending the ongoing nothingness that was growing within me. I think many people closest to me knew something was wrong but couldn't put their finger on it exactly, which I don't hold against them. I had become an expert at masking or hiding my mental ill health, even when I didn't know what depression or anxiety really was. Sure, I'd heard of it, but usually in a negative way, and what teen wants their peers to see that? Certainly not me. I even declined my mother's offer to take me to a therapist, insisting I was fine. It wasn't until I was eighteen that I had an honest conversation with myself about my mental health and took the first step in seeking help – seeing my doctor who prescribed me medication and then referred me to a therapist.

I wish my mental health journey improved from that moment on, that it had a nice ending wrapped in pretty paper and bows. It doesn't. Instead, I'd say my journey has had major highs and major lows. Some days are sunny, and others are full of dark clouds and rumbling thunder. For me, my depression has been cyclical, as if it has seasons attached to it. I will go months at a time without overwhelming thoughts or the unbearable weight of nothingness in my chest, then, just as it left, it will often return quickly and without warning. Though, at times, I can feel it coming on like the pain in an old man's bones when the weather turns sour – slow and building. There have been moments during my dark seasons that I've had a plan to end my life but was able to reach out to my therapist and several people within my incredible support system. Without these people and the tools my therapist has given me (along with prescription medication), I probably wouldn't be here typing this introduction today. Yet, that isn't the reality for so many across the world.

According to The WHO special initiative for mental health (2019-2023): universal health coverage for mental health[1], "more than 80% of people experiencing mental health conditions, including individuals experiencing neurological and substance use disorders, are without any form of quality, affordable mental health care." Looking more closely at the data, you'll find that, in 2017, an estimated 970 million people were living with a mental health condition or substance use disorder[2], and that number has increased by 13% as of 2022[3]. The initiative also reported that suicide mortality is high, accounting for close to 800,00 deaths per year, with those numbers accounting for the second leading cause of death among 15 to 29-year-olds. But it's not just young people being disproportionately affected, it's also those who live in poverty; those who live in low- and middle-income countries; those who are affected by humanitarian crises; and those affected by other forms of adversity. I'm no data scientist, but these numbers are concerning. We are in a global mental health crisis, and despite the number of initiatives out there, it never feels like enough is being done to relieve that crisis.

I believe that one of the main issues within all the numbers and statistics is just that – people are reduced to numbers and statistics. While there are more people using social media platforms such as Instagram and Twitter to voice their mental health experiences, so many mental health issues are spoken about in such a clinical way by journalists or by doctors or by organizations. Very rarely do we get the opportunity to hear mental health stories told by those who live with mental ill

1 World Health Organization. (2019). The WHO special initiative for mental health (2019-2023): universal health coverage for mental health. World Health Organization. https://apps.who.int/iris/handle/10665/310981.

2 Ritchie, Hannah. "Global Mental Health: Five Key Insights Which Emerge from the Data." *Our World in Data*, 16 May 2018, https://ourworldindata.org/global-mental-health.

3 "Mental Health." *World Health Organization*, https://www.who.int/health-topics/mental-health.

health daily. In part, this is due to the fear that comes with speaking one's truth. People shouldn't feel forced to share their stories and we, as humans, aren't obligated to share each tiny detail. I even edited down my own story into a bite sized version of its complexity. But another reason we don't hear these stories is that those suffering are often talked over and dismissed, as if mental health were nothing more than a papercut they must "get over" without complaint. Dismiss someone enough times and they are going to stop speaking all together. Remove their ability to speak up, and they become lost to the systems that do more harm than help.

Having been a solo advocate for mental health for years now, I felt compelled to bring together this anthology. I wanted to give others a platform to share their personal stories and to speak up about how mental health has affected their lives. In this anthology you'll find a profound group of authors whose experiences cover a broad range of lived experiences centered around mental ill health. Some will be difficult to navigate through, some will fill you with hope, all will broaden your understanding of what it means to live with mental ill health. These are their stories to tell without the hindrance of gatekeeping or overshadowing voices of doubt. If you are struggling with your own mental health, I hope you come away from this anthology knowing you aren't alone in your struggle. It is here, together, that we exchange our whispers for a roar and a right to be heard. It is here we fight for those who can't speak up. It is here we make mental health more than a buzzword – we make it a rallying cry for less stigma and more action, more change.

HANNAH FIELDS
Publisher/Founder
Folkways Press

NUT CLUSTER

by Hazel Norbury

A hazel can be a hard nut to crack, unless you're a squirrel, or you find a plier-style nutcracker languishing amongst your unused kitchen paraphernalia. Even if you do manage to crush the shell and the nut pops out unscathed, you wonder whether your efforts were worth it for such a small, hard blob. But if you're the owner of Ferrero Rocher, your endeavors are very much worth it, as his hazels are gathered into the bosom of his factory in Alba, Italy and subjected to a process so clandestine, no smart phones or notebooks are ever allowed to record what happens.

A bit like my life in therapy. Years of secret, die-of-shame outpourings in rooms uniformly furnished with a comfy chair, a cushion, and a potted plant. Psychosynthesis: two years. Full-time non-residential therapeutic community: three years. Psychodynamic group therapy: nine years. Women's survivors' groups: one year. Psychoanalytic therapy: six years. Plus, self-referrals to crisis residential services. Stays of up to four weeks, six times since the mid-nineties. If I'm not mistaken, that's around twenty years of therapy, at least half of it paid for by me. At the last estimate, close to £25,000.

"You managed to build a life for yourself before you became ill. That's why you're not traipsing through hospital corridors in your dressing gown," one practitioner said, as I railed against the "Why me?" "Why not you?" conundrum through a veil of bitter tears on the long road from victim to survivor.

Two decades of exposing the kernel of my experiences to realize the world owed me nothing.

The blank stare of the psychoanalytic therapist, the barely perceptible click of her clock ticking down the minutes as my unconscious thoughts embarked on their odyssey towards consciousness in the hope of releasing repressed emotion and experience: "Whenever we get near your trauma, you become unwell."

The raised, bushy brow of the psychosynthesis practitioner; the folds of her moss-green velour dress rippling with the flow of soul and spirit from the Self into all humanity: "I'm rather afraid of your anger."

The weary, nine-year smile of the group therapist swaddled in her mohair shawl, keen to divine the unconscious processes which informed my presenting behavior: "For some clients the *journey* will take a little longer."

The portly bartender of the pub beside the therapeutic community where we'd retreat most afternoons, wiping his hands on his apron: "Does she want another beer, the woman who cries?"

There's no doubt the work offered containment. Twenty years of hewing the raw slab into something more palatable. It kept the lid off the coffin and allowed me to flounder in my goo of shame and fear without drowning and, occasionally, studded my consciousness with tiny clusters of insight.

And for that I am grateful.

Does it even matter what has molded or shaped me, whether my outer shell is easily penetrated, and I can ooze with grief or crumble into despair, explode into tiny atoms of rage, as long as the image I present to the world is high quality and tastefully presented?

For me, it mattered. It wasn't enough to spend an hour a week submerged in a whirlpool of emotion or appreciating the influence of my early experiences on the development of my personality and behavior; plough through Freud, Alice Miller, Dorothy Rowe, R D Laing, Peter Levine, and others; head to three-hour evening classes in psychology after a day spent supporting homeless clients with drug, alcohol and, domestic violence issues.

There had to be something else I could do to *cure* myself. Out of therapy and into the mental health system? Maybe there was a wonder drug more effective than my anti-depressants? When I took voluntary redundancy from a housing charity in 2007 and got the first job I applied for, my GP was delighted. "Congratulations! A nationally advertised vacancy in the Guardian," she crowed. There would be no referrals to psychiatrists, no formal engagement with the 'system' for someone who was so obviously the gold-wrapped, morsel of perfection.

There came a point when I almost accepted my lot: that the most I could hope for was damage limitation. After all, everyone has their good and *not-so-good* days. Add on a flat, a job, empathetic colleagues and friends, enough money for food, alcohol and holidays abroad. Not forgetting my people-pleasing perfectionism which garnered my reputation as a hard-working, loyal employee.

Time to stop the self-indulgent rumination and get on with life.

So, at the age of fifty-two, I dispensed with therapy, tiptoed into the world, an unaccompanied minor, and explored new strategies for harnessing my emotions: boxing training, yoga, meditation, and sharing with those I judged able to tolerate distressing thoughts. Knowing the residential crisis house was there to catch me if I faltered enabled me to keep stumbling forward.

And then a miracle happened. I was bullied at work. The one place I'd always managed to distract myself from the chaos within. A three against one scenario. I didn't stand a chance. My GP, sensing an imminent catastrophe, referred me to a specialist NHS psychology service. That's how bullying became a blessing. After years serving an apprenticeship in psychodynamic and psychoanalytic therapy, the real work would begin. I would finally access my unconscious and uncover what was driving my deepest fears and longings. No more shouting into a void or dissolving into gloop. Instead, a tangible and methodical way of mapping my thought processes with defined and identifiable goals.

Fourteen months later I met my therapist, Joycelyn. Petite, blonde-haired, smocks and clogs. She explained how CBT trauma-focused therapy worked: stabilization, processing, and integration.

Trauma.

The word bounced off the wall and slammed into my face.

Jocelyn smiled. "It's ok, take your time," she said, as I flustered for a pen in my bag. "Where'd you go just now?"

I stared at her puzzled, not even aware I'd left, let alone where I'd gone to. She pointed to a couple of juggler-colored stress balls on the table in front of me and smiled. "How do they feel?"

I picked them up and squeezed. "Like a pair of bollocks," I said, as emotionless as a psychopath.

The following session the balls had disappeared, replaced by a succession of other grounding objects: keys, pebbles, and pinecones, which met the same fate. Eventually I settled on a lemon verbena candle, its sharp, sweet tang powerful enough to brighten the furthest reaches of my mind and wick me back to the present.

We admitted defeat on safe spaces and superheroes. I'd picture ornate gardens, tranquil lakesides, rugged mountain trails, but he'd always be there behind a tree or boulder playing peek-a-boo. I summoned Batman, the Terminator, a whole tribe of native American braves, the crowd at Anfield. To no avail.

At the start of the third session, Jocelyn handed me a book: *Coping with Trauma-Related Dissociation*, Boon, Suzette, et al. W.W Norton, 2011. The immediate sensation of someone else curtained behind my eyeballs reading the title. When I stashed it in my bag as if no-one were looking, Jocelyn laughed and said it was her office copy.

The A4-sized tome of 470 pages thudded through my letterbox. I ingested the contents in two sittings. After years of scrabbling for crumbs of insight, three practitioners I'd never met had allowed all five feet eleven of me to pour myself into the pages of their work in return for an explanation of who I was, why I was and what to do about it. It took a couple of weeks of perching precariously on the continuum of PTSD, complex PTSD, DDNOS (Dissociative Disorder Not Otherwise Specified) and DID (Dissociative Identity Disorder) for Jocelyn to assign me a diagnosis.

Complex PTSD.

Although no previous practitioner had mentioned the term, I'd always known my hypervigilance and murderous rage were markers of PTSD. This new diagnosis for those who have suffered repeated trauma enveloped me like a comfort blanket. The decades of flailing in the goo, my brain too overwhelmed by emotion to think rationally, were over. Here at last was an opportunity to take control of the parts of myself which had always controlled me. That's how one afternoon, with my candle and Jocelyn's presence for reassurance, I began taking slow and purposeful steps into my core.

No sooner had my eyes accustomed to the gloom than a terrified shrieking zig-zagged through the air as memory fragments stuck in trauma-time crashed around the space like frightened birds. The ground shook with the rage of my tormentor. Vivid flashbacks forked against the walls and splintered into shards of grief and shame. As decades of emotion shot through me, I felt myself disintegrating inside a kaleidoscope of my existence.

But with Jocelyn nearby and the scent of the candle clearing my head, I stood firm and anchored myself to the present. By learning to recognize the minutest shift in bodily sensation, identify the trigger and catch the thought before the emotion took hold, I managed to detach from the chaos and not get dragged in, first for seconds, then whole minutes. In a nutshell, I trained my brain to react differently.

Except fifteen sessions in, a huge, shaggy dog leapt out from a flashback. Rising up like a bear on its hind legs, saliva dripping from its maw, it knocked me backwards and into the cocoon of a crisis house where I sat in the art room cradling crayons and tears and allowed its canine image to streak the canvas. Five decades on and still new memories surfacing: it's the worst ones that stay hidden the longest. Jocelyn offered me an additional ten sessions, the last few strung out over three-week intervals.

Enveloped in a cloud of lemon verbena, I diligently practiced my skills for several weeks before the old patterns crept alongside the new. But the tools were there and became easier to use. I even struck up conversations with the dissociated parts of me. "Not today, thank you," I'd say, grannie-like, to the morning taunt from the critic who wanted me dead, rather than reacting with a torrent of fucks and c-bombs. "Just acknowledge his presence, allow him to be there," Jocelyn had said.

She'd suggested a year for the work to settle, after which I tried to find private, trauma-focused practitioners to begin the next stage. The cost was upwards of £120 per session and double for processing. The profile of an ex-GP turned therapist looked promising and I visited her office in London Bridge twice. But my anxiety about the thin, grubby walls adjoining a busy reception and spending upwards of an estimated £3,000 on a block of twenty sessions drove my trauma so far underground the sessions became pointless. My GP agreed to a second referral to the NHS.

"So nice to see you again. You look really well," Claire, my assessor, said.

I braced myself for what was coming. "We normally only offer one bite of the cherry."

The cyanide in the pip was already leaking out. "But I haven't done any processing work," I said. "It took the full six months to stabilize."

Claire shrugged. "Any CBT therapist can do processing."

"I tried. It didn't work. I need a safe space. I can't afford that kind of money."

Their system had changed. If accepted, I'd attend a group for eight weeks first to explore common themes such as anger, fear, relationships, and concepts like the window of tolerance and fight, flight, and freeze responses. The invitation to join the waiting list arrived two days later. Six months on, seven women and I sat clutching pinecones and sniffing essential oils in a room which bore witness to an average of five decades each of unprocessed trauma: more than four hundred years, which overwhelmed three of the group into leaving. The rest of us had just begun to bond and open up about our daily struggles to live with trauma when the group finished.

Three months became six, then seven, through spring, summer and into autumn. The promise of individual sessions shriveled like the leaves on the trees. Until September 2020, when Karen's black bob, T-bar heels, and flouncy blouses swished along the corridor towards me. She sparkled with wit and intelligence, her champagne glass always half full in a sod-the-calories type of way. Five sessions in preparation for processing, each began with stabilization, followed by a detailed explanation of what processing would entail.

That was my first encounter with EMDR (Eye Movement Desensitization and Re-processing) as a tool for accessing my unprocessed trauma memories. A light bar provided a socially distanced alternative to Karen's two fingers. An ascent into *Game of Thrones*, I watched myself ride magic carpets and stallions through bizarre, full-color representations of my life. In every scene my abuser played a starring role – snake charmer, travelling salesman, bartender. I shot him in the head and splattered his brain, melted him in a pizza oven, flung him into the jaws of a crocodile, hacked him into dog food with a machete, but each time he reformed out of the gore into a slime of slugs tonguing towards me.

I remember walking back to the overground in a daze. I'd always known I'd internalized my abuser, turning his hatred against myself, but to learn I co-existed with an indestructible assassin was truly shocking.

It took three processing sessions to empty my unconscious and a fourth one to embed a blueprint for the ideal me, the me who would have fought back, would have called the police, would have asserted herself.

"EMDR is definitely the one for you," Karen said. "You work so hard. You read the books. You engage with the process."

"I have to," I said. "I just want to understand."

"But what we really need is for you to connect the words to the emotion. There's something I want to try next week."

Our penultimate session offered me the chance to meet him: not the eighty-six-year-old man who still lives in North Wales, but the younger, stronger, sadist.

"What would you want to say to him. Imagine he's sitting right there?"

She pointed to an empty chair, just to my right. My gaze travelled over the tatty cushion and spindly legs.

"I'd want to tell him to fuck off," I said.

"So, go on, tell him to, let rip."

I felt it rising. My revulsion. Like a pan of sour milk about to boil over. The froth of gentle bubbles which ran up the sides, words then phrases forming in the momentum. Faster and faster until they hurled themselves over the edge.

"Die, you bastard! Fuck off and die!" I lunged at the chair and smashed it at the wall, shattering its legs into splinters, bones protruding from flesh, my throat scorched with fire.

Except my feet never left the ground.

"Impressive," said Karen. "Now imagine you're much younger. What would he say to the child you sitting there?"

She was five with shoulder-length, sleek waves, and an impish smile. Her legs dangled mid-way to the floor.

"You should have died in the womb. You weren't meant to live. Paul died and then you arrived. A girl. A mistake."

The little girl's cheeks whitened with fear.

"What would you say back?"

I shook my head. I had no words, but my arms went round her.

"Does he want to say anything?" Karen asked.

The words from my mouth as puzzling as they were unexpected. "I don't know how else to be."

"Interesting," Karen said. "Why not tell him how you'd like him to behave. Try and reach a compromise."

"It's too late," I said. "He'll never change. He'll always want me dead."

Karen crossed her arms. “So, you need to challenge him,” she said. “Be calm. Be assertive. Let’s do a role play. I’ll be him.”

Role play? She was the one on a roll. But I couldn’t let her down. One of the only therapists who pushed beyond containment. She wanted something different for me.

“You’re just a waste of space.”

I realized in an instant the empty chair work had been the warm-up as well as a risk assessment. “Is that so?” Ugly fuck.

“You don’t deserve anything good in your life.”

“Neither do you.” Idiot fuck.

“You’re not worth it.”

“And I suppose you are.” Pointless fuck.

“I’m more intelligent than you.”

“With that amoeba intellect.” Thick fuck. “And you’re just an arsehole.” A fucking arsehole.

Karen’s hand flew to her mouth. “You called me an arsehole.”

She tossed her head back and roared with laughter. “You called me an arsehole.”

A fucking arsehole. “I enjoyed it.”

“Get lost.”

“No, you get lost.” Fucking arsehole.

We both doubled up and, for a moment, I tasted the nut cluster of life in all its crack and crunch. After so many years of silence – family, work, self-imposed – I savored the sound as much as the taste.

These days we spar too, him and I, over coffee. He takes it black with two sugars. It’s not the coffee he likes best, though. His eyes glow at the sight of the neat rows of gold, foil-wrapped chocolate. I nudge the tray towards him, and he grabs one, tears off the wrapping and swallows it whole, as though if he didn’t someone might snatch it from him.

My turn and I lift a chocolate out of its groove, carefully removing the paper case and wrapping.

"If you take your time with it," I say, "you can appreciate all the layers."

He stares with uncertainty and embarrassment, like a child who's misbehaved, and, in his vulnerability, I see a way for us to cohabit. That I can separate the eighty-six-year-old who'd sit slightly off camera at the weekly online family quiz from the man who stole a childhood.

Apart from the final few, most of my sessions with Karen were in person, squeezed between COVID-19 lockdowns. I emailed her a fictionalized account of one of my EMDR experiences as a thank you.

"We're no longer offering one-to-ones, only groups," she said, on our last Zoom call. "We're simply overwhelmed. You've been lucky."

I try not to think about those who haven't been so lucky: their pre-pandemic ascent up the waiting lists for one-to-one support obliterated, and the scores of traumatized NHS, care home staff and families torn apart by COVID-19. Not to mention those facing the poverty of heat or eat in our broken economy. How will they survive, how will we all survive, in a world full of unprocessed trauma?

As for me, I'm still not *cured*. That destination will always be out of reach. But, in the last few years, with the benefit of specialist support, I've travelled further towards self-acceptance and recovery than ever before.

Call me old-fashioned, but I'm not quite ready for ayahuasca ceremonies in the Amazonian jungle. I'll stick with EMDR. But, barring the financial means to pay for more sessions, or a mental health catastrophe which catapults me straight onto an NHS waiting list, this part of my journey's over.

Did all those sessions of traditional therapy enable me to make better use of trauma-informed treatment when I was finally offered the opportunity? Or, had CBT and EMDR modalities been available in the early nineties, could I have achieved comparable results in a fraction of the time and saved myself thousands of pounds? Whatever the truth, I did the best I could with the resources I had: physical and mental as well as financial. And that's all I can ever do.

Bio: Hazel lives in London and works in a university. After years in the creative wilderness, she's currently doing a part-time MA in Creative Writing and, second time around, is really enjoying being a student.

JOINING THE THERAPEUTIC COMMUNITY:

HOW GROUP THERAPY HELPED MY MENTAL HEALTH

by Katie Kent

A few years ago, as I lay crying on my bed after a friendship had ended, having taken a few pills, and fighting suicidal thoughts, it seemed that my life would never get better. I'd been suffering with mental illness for most of my life, but I was in a particularly bad period at that moment.

In my earlier life, I had struggled with anorexia and social anxiety, but in my 30s I was diagnosed with both Obsessive Compulsive Disorder (OCD) and Borderline Personality Disorder (BPD). Looking back, these diagnoses made sense considering some of my behaviors as a teenager and in my 20s.

My OCD was focused mainly around "rules" that my brain told me I had to follow. Over the years, these rules affected my life to a great degree – affecting my study at university, my work, eating habits, personal relationships, and even my hobbies. My anorexia began when I read something about how much fat people should be eating and about the dangers of being overweight – leading to the typical OCD pattern of an obsession (I might get fat, therefore becoming unhealthy and undesirable to other people) and compulsions (I must count the fat in everything I eat; I must stick to a fixed, low amount of fat every day; there are certain foods I can never eat as they are too fattening).

My brain screamed at me to follow the rules; if I didn't, the obsession I feared might come true. This pattern was repeated in many areas of my life. For example, at university I was sure I would fail if I didn't study at least three hours a day, and that would ruin my life. I'd time my study obsessively. In my 30s, the health obsession came back with a vengeance after one of the staff at my local gym told me I should be exercising 2.5 hours a week. I also got a fitness tracker and fixated on making sure I achieved 10,000 steps per day. These are usually healthy behaviors, but my brain turned them into unhealthy ones as I became obsessive over them. At work, I stressed that I was going to run out of work in the future and get fired, so I'd stockpile emails, too scared to answer them all in case they ran out, which often left me behind on my work.

My BPD also affected my life in many ways. I often formed intense attachments with people who showed me sympathy and care. These people weren't just friends; I clearly saw them as replacement parental figures and looked to them to 'fix' me. Instead, a few years on, none of these people talk to me anymore, having ended the friendships because it became too intense for them. I'd talk about myself and my problems all the time, subconsciously thinking that this would keep people from leaving me, as they'd feel sorry for me. Fear of abandonment is one of the main BPD traits, and it affected me greatly. When these friendships ended, it just reinforced all the horrible things I thought about myself, and I'd reach out for someone new to replace them. It became a vicious cycle.

Self-hatred ruled my existence, and my self-esteem was almost non-existent. I'd berate myself often, whether I deserved it or not, and wrote a "diary" which consisted of me telling myself how horrible and worthless I was, and how people didn't care about me and that I deserved to die. I think this self-hatred was why I became so attached to people. I used them to measure my self-worth. I'd worry about my wife and friends leaving me all the time, which seemed like the worst fate ever – without them, what was the point of me being alive?

I'd also get very jealous over other people receiving any attention, positive or negative. If someone else was praised for something, I'd feel like people were saying that they were brilliant, and I was useless. If someone was struggling with something and people showed sympathy towards them, it would feel like people were saying they cared about them and didn't care about me. I remember once having two friends over who both had physical health problems, and as I listened to them talking to each other about these illnesses and showing each other sympathy, I felt like I'd been stabbed in the gut. I wanted to say, "What about me?" It felt like I didn't matter. Sometimes this feeling would cause me to reach out and compete for attention, and sometimes I'd just revert to the quiet self-hatred and negative diary entries.

Another BPD trait that has affected me, and that was tied into the things I've described above, was changeable emotions. I could be having a good day, but if someone I felt attached to took a while to reply to one of my messages or said the 'wrong' thing, or if I witnessed someone else receiving attention, my mood would plummet and I'd suddenly feel rubbish and descend into self-hatred. This pattern could happen many times in a day and was exhausting for both me and the people around me. It could be triggered by the simplest things, such as my wife telling me I had loaded the dishwasher incorrectly or a friend saying they were going out and wouldn't be able to reply to me until the next day.

BPD is the only mental illness where self-harm and suicidal thoughts are one of the diagnostic criteria. I really struggled with this one, descending into suicidal fantasies whenever I felt criticized or rejected. Unlike many people with BPD, I didn't come close to acting on my suicidal ideation – the small overdoses I took, one in my early 20s and one in my late 30s when my friend left me, were both intended as cries for help. I did, however, harm myself by cutting quite often. My self-harm was mostly to punish myself and was tied in with my self-hatred.

My OCD and BPD may seem like separate, distinct mental illnesses, but they did overlap. One of my OCD obsessions revolved around feeling like I needed to sleep with my wife once a week, the consequence of which my brain told me was that we would break up otherwise, which came from my fear of abandonment. When my OCD was particularly bad, especially concerning my relationship and my job, the self-harm urges, and suicidal thoughts struck with a vengeance. And I think my need for attention and care, stemming from my BPD, subconsciously made my OCD worse as I was scared by the thought of losing my OCD – who would care about me if I wasn't sick?

Therapy has changed me for the better. It's taught me that I won't necessarily ever "cure" my mental illnesses, but that they can be managed, and has given me the tools to do that. I started by paying to see a private therapist – not cheap, but she was knowledgeable, sympathetic, and helped me when I was feeling at my worst. It was her who diagnosed me with BPD. I do wonder, though, whether the excessive focus on me that naturally came from private therapy did sometimes reinforce my need for attention.

I was given the maximum number of Cognitive Behavior Therapy (CBT) sessions provided by the NHS. My NHS therapist was understanding and helpful, and I managed to make progress on some of my obsessive behaviors, like avoiding timing my walking, but I found it very difficult to tackle some of the harder obsessions around sex, exercise, and work, for example.

Group therapy is what I've found the most useful for me. Nearly three years ago I finally came to the top of the waiting list with the Complex Needs Service – a personality disorder service that organizes and runs the therapy groups – and was referred for an assessment. My assessor was kind and knowledgeable, asking me about my childhood and the thoughts and behaviors that I struggled with. Because of my need for attention, I was always worried that there was nothing really wrong with me – maybe I was just a selfish person – and that I didn't deserve help, but as soon as I started to describe my problems with relationships he told me immediately that he knew that I had come to the right place. He backed up my earlier diagnosis of BPD after I completed a personality disorders questionnaire.

After my assessment I went back onto a short waiting list, but before too long, my name came to the top, and I started in ESG (the Emotional Skills Group) – a short group that met once a week for a couple of hours and aimed to teach skills to help us deal with our emotions. This group introduced me to some therapeutic concepts and to the idea of group therapy, allowing me to settle in and feel like I belonged. Part of the discussions in the group were also focused on moving onto the next stage, the Therapeutic Community (TC), and members of that group visited our group every week so that we could get to know them. After about six months I felt ready to move on, and visited the TC to present my case conference and my application to join, which is a set of questions about our issues and what we want to work on and how we feel the TC can help us. I was voted in unanimously and began TC in October 2019. TC is usually an 18-month program, but when COVID-19 struck, our time was extended by six months as we weren't able to meet, instead receiving weekly phone calls from the therapists in the group. After that time, we moved onto meeting online over Zoom, which continues to this day.

Being in the ESG and then the TC has really helped me with my mental health in a few ways. Firstly, it's brought me a sense of belonging that I didn't always feel before. Before I joined ESG I didn't know anyone else with a personality disorder. Being around other people with similar problems to mine meant that I had like-minded people who often struggled with the same things that I did, and it really felt like a community as we offered support to each other. The validation I've received from the group is something I had been searching for all my life – much of my behavior had been misunderstood by other people, who just saw me as attention-seeking or as someone who constantly overreacted. It's also helped me relate to others outside the group in healthier ways. I've realized that people do care about me and that them not responding to something I've said in a certain way doesn't mean that they hate me or don't want to know me.

Part of the TC that most people find difficult is the support call system. We have each other's phone numbers and are encouraged to reach out to other members if we are struggling or want to talk over an issue or feeling or even celebrate a success. In my case, I have found this difficult because of my need for attention, so I worried I would become reliant on this, but that hasn't been the case. We are required to discuss everything that happens in the calls in our group sessions, reporting every week on who we have called and what the conversations were about. Through the calls I have been offered new ways to think about things I've struggled with, been challenged in healthy ways on things I've said or thought, and built up relationships with group members, who I hope will become friends once we've left the group.

Finally, the therapists and other TC members have also helped me explore the reasons for my thoughts, feelings and behaviors, and to practice healthier behavior and responses instead. In the past I'd felt guilty when I'd heard other people with BPD talking about their experiences of abuse and other childhood traumas – I'd not experienced anything like that – but the group made me realize that the death of my baby brother when I was three years old was no less traumatic than other sufferers' childhoods. This realization has lessened some of the feelings of guilt I felt often about everyday things. Exploring how I felt about his death has helped me to finally grieve for him, almost 40 years later. With the group's support, I even plucked up the courage to ask my parents about the circumstances around his death, which I couldn't remember and had been afraid to ask about in case it upset them. This conversation gave me some answers that I had always wondered about and let me see how this event affected my childhood and the development of my BPD and OCD. Questioning why something had triggered me by talking about it in the group has helped me recognize my triggers more easily before they affect my behavior, or at least question my responses.

The therapists have introduced us to therapeutic concepts that have contributed to my understanding of my own illnesses. Two of the most relevant to me have been the drama triangle and the PAC (parent, adult, child) model. The drama triangle is formed of three people – persecutor, victim, and rescuer. I realized that throughout much of my life I've taken the role of victim, whereas others I have become attached to have tried to rescue me. The group has shown me how I can step out of the drama triangle and adopt a healthier role in my relationships. The PAC model is similar to the drama triangle, but instead the roles are parent, adult, and child. Through exploring this model I've realized that I've been constantly adopting the child role in my relationships, wanting others to parent me. This has helped me practice how to be an adult in my relationships, relating to others also as adults rather than expecting them to look after me, therefore forcing them into a parent role.

As I prepare to leave the TC in two months, I want to revisit the main symptoms of my mental illnesses and how therapy has helped with them. It was only recently that I felt able to challenge the rules that my OCD set for me around measuring, counting, and timing things. This is likely to be something I struggle with for the rest of my life to an extent, but I've made some progress with some of my obsessive behaviors. I was on a therapeutic agreement recently, deciding to practice being more spontaneous and to resist some of the rules. With the support of the TC, I've mixed up my exercise routine, skipped a walk if I haven't felt up to it or have been busy with something else, and done things without planning them. I still feel anxious when I have few emails at work, but I've been working on challenging myself and getting through them despite feeling that anxiety.

It's been a while since I had an obsessive attachment with a friend – there have been people at work I've been close to, and I've been upset when they've left work, but these friendships feel a lot healthier. We are still friends, and I don't feel the need to have their attention all the time. My relationship with my wife has gotten better, too – I used to worry constantly that she would leave me, and this affected my behavior with her, but I don't worry about that anywhere as much as I used to. I don't feel the need to tell everyone when I'm feeling bad in order to get that care I had desperately been searching for my entire life.

I'm not sure I can ever say that I love myself, but at least I like myself now. The negative thoughts towards myself sometimes creep in, but they are not pervasive like they used to be. I'm capable of seeing my good points, and although I have struggled with loneliness lately, I don't feel like I need to measure my self-worth through other people's feelings about me.

The jealousy that I used to feel when someone else received attention has not completely gone and, again, is likely to be something I continue to struggle with. However, I am now able to see someone else receive sympathy without feeling that overwhelming jealousy. I worried that being around other 'sick' people in the TC would trigger my jealousy when they talked about their own thoughts and feelings and received sympathy, but instead it has taught me how to be more tolerant of other people's difficulties without feeling jealous.

My changeable emotions came from my triggers, and triggers will always be there, but therapy has helped me recognize my triggers and think about my reactions towards them. It's helped me stop and think about how I'm feeling before I react to them in a certain way.

I haven't self-harmed since I started in TC as it's one of the rules of the group, and if we break it, we're expected to be honest about that and discuss with the group why we did it and what the ramifications should be. There have been times when I have had strong urges to do it, and the knowledge that I would have to discuss it with everyone has put me off. I thought that once I left TC, I wouldn't be able to resist as easily because I wouldn't have to report it back, but now I feel that even without that, it's a behavior that I don't want to go back to. I don't need it. I don't need to punish myself. The suicidal thoughts haven't entirely left me, but they don't permeate every aspect of my life like they used to.

I don't consider myself "cured," but I can certainly manage my illnesses a lot better than before I started group therapy. It's not been easy at times, and I've had to push myself to challenge old thoughts and behaviors, but I am ready to leave the group. I feel I have the tools I need to live my life in a healthy way and without needing that professional support for the first time in years. Group therapy can work, and I've seen that in the people who left the TC before me, as well as in myself.

Bio: Katie Kent is a writer living in the UK with her wife, cat and dog. She likes to write stories, mostly YA, about LGTBQ characters, mental illness, time travel and the future – sometimes all in the same story! Her fiction has been published in *Youth Imagination*, *Limeoncello* and *Flash Fiction Magazine*, amongst others, and in anthologies including *The Trouble with Time Travel*, *Summer of Speculation: Catastrophe*, *Growth* and *My Heart to Yours*. Her non-fiction, mostly mental health-related, is published in *The Mighty*, *You & Me Magazine*, *Ailment*, *OC87 Recovery Diaries* and *Feels Zine*. Her website is at https://www.katiekentwriter.com/.

YOUR STAY IN LONG RIVER PSYCHIATRIC HOSPITAL:

A GUIDE

by Liz Whittaker

INTRODUCTION

Welcome to Long River Psychiatric Hospital. We're so glad you've taken this important step in your mental health journey. This guide will help you understand what to expect during your stay with us and will answer any questions you may have.

A note on budget and patient safety: A psychiatric hospital may feel like something between a prison and a poorly funded summer camp. The hallways are all linoleum, and if there is carpet, it will be that industrial style that will make the whole place feel like a dorm room. There will be nothing comforting in the aesthetics of this place. Your room will have battered oak furniture, a scuffed trash can, and a mattress that resembles a gym mat. While you may not find these amenities as comfortable, please note that everything has been curated for patient safety. No doors may be locked at any time, and the shape of the door handles prevent anything being attached to them. The shower curtain is a heavy industrial fabric, which cannot be folded, twisted, or ripped. There are no plastic bags anywhere in the space, including in trash cans. If you wish to decorate your space, you may use a small amount of tape (available at the nurse's station) to post art made during recreation therapy.

POSSIBLE REASONS FOR ADMITTING YOURSELF

Perhaps the seeds of anxiety and depression blossomed within you long ago. You've had your dose of Zoloft, your years of cognitive-behavioral therapy, and your coping mechanisms. But maybe on an evening in February, your husband will take your hands and calmly tell you that he doesn't want to be married to you anymore. He will move out within hours. A week later, he will sit next to you in a therapist's office with his fists clenched, sobbing about how the things you've done and not done have permanently damaged him. Perhaps you will hold in a scream until you get into your car, where it will tear through your throat as you bang the steering wheel. You will scrape the driver's side door on a concrete column as you speed away.

And it will hurt and hurt and hurt, and it will feel like the hurt will never end – and you will keep thinking about the bottles of pills in the medicine cabinet or the crunch of metal on a highway or a car left running in the garage. It will feel impossible to keep living this way, with this pain that doesn't end, that nothing fixes, that nothing eases. So, at 10 pm one night, you will drive yourself to Long River Psychiatric Hospital and tell them you need help.

THE ADMITTING PROCESS

This will take several hours and will include everything from questionnaires to urine tests. You will also be strip searched, which will be less traumatic than you think. There will be no invasive gloved fingers. You will strip down to nothing, and the nurses will tell you to stand with your feet wider than shoulder-width apart. You will then be asked to squat quickly. Until that moment, it will never have occurred to you how impossible it would be to keep anything hidden in any body cavity while squatting quickly. Even in your distress, there will be a corner of your mind that will think, "Well, now I've done a strip search." Your belongings will be subject to a search as well, and anything potentially dangerous will be confiscated (see the next section for a list of dangerous items).

ITEMS NOT ALLOWED IN THE WARD

Bras with underwires are considered dangerous and are not permitted. You must either remove the wires, go without a bra, or use a wireless one.

Non-spiritual literature is prohibited, unless approved by a therapist. You may possibly get a novel (Valerie Martin's *Mary Reilly*) through the doors, because the admitting nurses think it looks harmless. You will be extremely grateful for this over the next few days.

Toiletries of any kind are not allowed, including Chapstick. Shampoo and soap will be dispensed in paper condiment cups at the nurse's station right before use. You may request Vaseline for chapped lips and hand lotion for dry skin, if necessary.

Cell phones must be surrendered.

Pens, pencils, or other writing utensils will be confiscated. You will be provided with crayons or golf pencils if you need to write anything down. You will come to miss writing with a pen more than you ever thought possible.

Shoelaces, belts, jewelry, watches, and hair ties must be removed.

Your personal journal must remain locked away. Instead, you will be provided with a wide-ruled composition notebook. This will annoy you at first, but later, you will come to appreciate how your time in the hospital is kept and contained in these unique pages.

Suitcases, purses, or plastic bags are all prohibited. Any of your belongings that make it past screening will be placed in a paper bag and handed to you.

AFTER ADMISSION

You will spend much of the first day lying in bed, sobbing uncontrollably, whispering, "Help me, somebody help me – please, please, please."

And it will feel like no one is helping you. No one will be there to hold you, comfort you, hand you pills that fix it all. The pain you were trying to ease will not be eased. It will continue to hurt. It will not be immediately and completely all better.

Your roommate for the first night will be a woman named Trisha, who will speak kind words and hand you pages of her artwork—pages colored in crayon—before she leaves. She will recognize what she is giving you as handfuls of hope, and you will feel that they are impossible to hold.

THE DAILY SCHEDULE

7:30 AM — Breakfast. Which is too early, especially when the lights in the hallway are never turned off, and your door is cracked open once per hour for bed/safety checks throughout the night. For this meal and all others, you and the other patients will gather by the door to the hallway, next to the nurse's station. Once everyone's name is marked off on a clipboard, a nurse will walk you through a series of doors that must be unlocked with a keycard, until you reach the cafeteria. The food will be of the same quality as those terrible elementary school cafeteria lunches you thought you had put behind you forever, though you can tell the woman behind the counter is trying. Chicken nuggets and soggy crinkle fries. Frozen things heated up again. You will have half an hour to eat.

8:00 AM — Morning meds dispensed.

9:00 AM — Recreation therapy. This will not seem to differ from other types of therapy, except for sometimes there's an activity involved, instead of just talking.

10:30 AM — Group therapy, during which one of a rotating cast of therapists will guide the group through ideas of stress management, addiction triggers, affirmations, and codependency. Words from therapists will be interspersed with non-sequiturs from patients. During a conversation about tools to handle stress, one patient will say, "This is just one planet, guys. I do this all the time." Another will ask, "Have you ever tasted dead lips?"

11:30 AM — Lunch. The same routine as breakfast.

1:00 PM — More group therapy. For the first few days, you will feel very strongly that none of this applies to you, that all of these people have problems that simply aren't the same as yours—addiction, miscarriages, borderline personality disorder, severe psychosis, etc. You are not one of these people, and this is not helping.

2:30 PM — Afternoon meds dispensed. At some point later in the afternoon, you'll have a one-on-one meeting with a therapist. They will make notes in an enormous binder that has your name on it. You will wonder how they could possibly have that big of a binder for you when you've been here less than a week.

5:00 PM — Dinner. See routine for all meals.

8:00 PM — Evening meds dispensed.

Between these activities, or if you choose to abstain from them, there is very little to do. You will spend much of your time sleeping, crying in your room, reading, and writing in your composition notebook. Towards the end of your stay, you will feel brave enough to go into the common room to watch television with the other patients. There will be a night when you all watch American Ninja Warrior together. Average people doing impossible things. Things that are impossible, but they're doing them anyway.

LIVING WITH OTHER PATIENTS

You will be sharing your experience with a number of other patients. Examples of the people you may encounter include:

Sam. A "fully enlightened" young man, obsessed with war. Mid-twenties. Manic, delusional, psychotic. He will explain that the gold on the top of the pyramids jammed radio signals and it overloaded the system and it caused 9/11. He will also tell a questionable story about a conversation he had with "Krishna." ("I said, 'Krishna. I am the embodiment of trust.' And he said, 'I will give you three queens.' I said, 'Krishna. I cannot please three women. A 17-year-old woman can't handle a 25-year-old man.' So, he gave me Parvati, who is now sealed in Shiva. I am so hungry.") There will also be moments when his free-flowing words will border on poetic. His description of a government building will sound like the work of Allen Ginsberg: "Scientifically backflip. Interchangeable locks. Floor after floor after floor. Complex camera systems. Free cigarettes."

Timothy. An elderly man there to detox. Strong southern accent and wet wracking cough. He will rarely come to the cafeteria for meals but will often request that someone bring him back some juice with Coke in it.

Mariah. Highly mercurial — sometimes kind and warm, sometimes angry and violent. Chronically dishonest. Interactions with her will remind you vaguely of being in middle school. Early thirties, but she seems younger. At one point, you will complain of your uterus hurting, and she will ask, in complete seriousness, "What's a uterus?"

Amy. A woman in her forties with long blonde hair that she often keeps in two buns on the top of her head. She lost her baby in a miscarriage a few weeks before. She is tall and kind and maternal, and some mornings you will watch her go still with pleasure as she drinks coffee and smokes a cigarette.

George. Early twenties. A homeless man who will sleep most of the time. Diabetic. Towards the end of your stay, he will intentionally get into a fist fight with another patient to prove that he "wasn't ready" to be released, in order to have access to a warm bed and insulin for a few more nights.

Leah. A woman in her sixties, with very long curly hair that is grey at the roots and brown at the tips. Paranoid, delusional. She will throw away all of her toiletries on a daily basis, and request new ones afterwards. She will speak in a constant, monotone, negative run-on sentence, starting at 5 am and not stopping until midnight or so, often walking relentlessly up and down the hall. (Example: "*That's why we have so many numbers in catalogs, numbers N.O. the abbreviation, because it's information overload on their parts, that's why we're all shooting up with heroin, and I've seen those cameras, they've been on the whole time, aimed right at everyone's crotches, but the only way to do detective work is by staying in the background and I stay in the background because I'm a prayer and not a drug dealer, that's just rude and it's a snap and that's how I'm training my cat, with snaps, so I never have to raise a hand to that fucking cat, but I'm tired of talking in riddles and I sound crazy but I'm not I just have too much confidential information in my head, you know, like postal workers, you know, in some countries, they don't even get mail except once a month and if I knew I'd be making a speech, I would have made another outline.*")

Luke. He will be the sanest person there, and he will only be there briefly. In his thirties, he is handsome in a sexy, dark kind of way. He will be hospitalized because of a bad drug trip. You will hear him talking on the nurse station phone to his friends. ("All that shit that John was saying? That wasn't real?") He will seem so lost, but will make phone call after phone call, apologizing and explaining, before leaving.

Alexis. She will be your roommate for most of your stay, and you will bond over a shared love of Harry Potter, and eventually you'll be for her what Trisha was for you.

Rob. He will come halfway through your stay. He is kind and funny, a hippie at heart in every sense. In his forties or fifties. He will crack jokes in group therapy to keep the mood light, and will often bring food back from the cafeteria. He may possibly be manic, but one day during group therapy, he will remind everyone in the group to "keep your head and your ass in the same room," and it will resonate so much with you that you will paint it and put it on your wall later.

TREATMENT COMPLETION

At some point, something will shift. Without much to distract you, you will have to just sit there and sort through your shit all at once. It will be the worst emotional pain of your life, condensed into a few days, in rooms where you couldn't hurt yourself in your attempt to escape it. There will be no choice but to heal, with meds and meetings and group therapy and sleep and routine.

And you'll start to see how little separates us from each other. You will sit in group therapy sessions and suddenly it will apply to you. You'll sit with the others at lunch, in the common room. At dinner one evening, an elderly woman from another ward will join your table and explain how she got through fentanyl detox by wheeling her wheelchair up and down the hallway all night until the pains were gone. When you tell her why you came to Long River Hospital, she'll nod sympathetically, then smile warmly at you and say "You'll be jest fine. I can tell jest by looking at ya."

By Friday night, you will feel a little bit of the sunshine that you thought was out of your reach forever. It won't fill you up completely, but it will be there. The hope that Trisha handed you when you arrived will start to wrap itself around your heart. You'll hand some of that hope to your new roommate Alexis, and you will see how she feels it is impossible to hold, like you felt when Trisha handed it to you. You trust that Alexis' heart will learn to carry it soon, like yours did.

DISCHARGE AND TRANSITIONING BACK TO NORMAL LIFE

Your father will pick you up late on a Saturday morning and will present you with a giant teddy bear when you meet him in the lobby. He will take you to lunch at Smashburger, and after days of hospital food, it will be the most indescribably delicious meal you have ever tasted in your entire life.

Leaving the hospital will feel like walking a long distance after having a bad flu. A remaining emotional soreness, an ache that reminds you to not rush, to take moments to just sit and be still. This stillness is one of the things you learned in the hospital, because you had no choice. Without to-do lists and Facebook and school to distract you, you found that you simply had to be still. When there's nothing else to notice, you notice the colors of the walls, the temperature in the room, the sounds humming quietly in the background. You'll take this skill of noticing with you when you leave.

You will keep a sense of connectedness after you leave. The woman experiencing homelessness on the corner could easily be your roommate at the hospital. The man ranting on the train station platform could be someone you sat next to at lunch, staying in another ward down the hall at Long River.

The only words to describe this belief are trite, but you will understand how little separates all of us.

You will press your hospital ID bracelet into the pages of your journal, and slowly work your way through the calls and emails and texts you've missed. You'll wash the dishes you left in the sink at your apartment. You'll do a load of laundry. You'll write with a pen.

You will probably still cry every single day for the next several months. But you will find ways to be still, to let the pain course through you and then away. You'll have moments of panic, and moments when you remind yourself to keep your head and your ass in the same room.

You'll be still.

You'll keep living.

Bio: Liz Whittaker received her MFA in Writing from Lindenwood University in 2017, and has been sharing essays, poems, and other work on her blog *She May Be Naked But She's Not Stupid* (https://butshesnotstupid.blogspot.com/) since 2004.

INHERITANCE

by Jess Witkins

When I was a child, my favorite game to play was a game I called "Orphan." The goal was to move around my house as long as I could without someone spotting me, which truth be told, wasn't that hard. As the much younger, youngest of four I wasn't really on anyone's radar. I'd steal food from the pantry, creep upstairs to my lair, a make-believe bunker I'd made by hanging string and old scarves from my dresser to a plant stand. I would stay there for hours, just me and my trusty stuffed animal cat, Caramel, whose fur was deeply matted.

Orphan was a game inspired more by Disney movies (*Toby Tyler, Pollyanna, Aladdin*) than by my actual childhood. For one, according to Disney, being an orphan meant I could talk to animals, and that sounded pretty cool. But because my parents were older than most other parents of kids my age, I developed anxiety that they wouldn't live to see me grow up. I think playing Orphan was just me casting myself as a survivor.

Christmas dinner with my family. 2019. We were at my sister's house, and we're all grown now, some with kids of their own. My parents, thankfully, both still with us. My sister has hidden conversation starters underneath everyone's plates and we go around the table answering questions. My father takes his turn.

"What is your happiest childhood memory?"

He answers.

"I must have been nine, or eleven maybe. I don't remember what the occasion was, but the whole family went out to eat. I ordered a hamburger, and it was the first time I'd ever been to a restaurant."

My siblings and I are stunned. Our father owned and ran a restaurant for over 20 years. We grew up bussing tables, eating last, and eating what was left on the buffet. We grew up in a restaurant. He remembers the first time he visited one.

We sat around a table full of Christmas goodies. Steaks for whoever wanted one. Roast pheasant, too.

"We were too poor to eat out," my father says.

My father's mother, my Grandma Marion, grew up very poor. She was one of three girls living in a dirt floor home. Her mother died when she was young, and my grandmother and her sisters were shuffled from relative to relative. Sometimes they couldn't go together.

Much of my grandmother's childhood was spent feeling unwanted, and she carried that feeling of burden into her marriage despite its longevity.

When my Grandma Marion was little, her favorite thing to do was sit on a chair in the kitchen, watching the mice in their home scurry up the pipes.

As an old woman, she took pride in her collection of fur coats – rabbit hair, I think. They were an impractical belonging for life in an old farmhouse and did not match the housecoats she wore or the curlers in her hair, but they were the invisible line marking, to her, that she'd "made it."

***

In college, I work as a desk attendant and housekeeper in the dorms. I pull other people's hair from drains. Once, I am asked to clean up vomit that has dried for days in a locked bathroom stall. I do it, crawling under the door to get in.

After that, I move into an apartment with three other girls. My mother keeps buying me plastic cups because one of the girls steals our dishes and puts them in bins we can see through but denies she has even used them.

I work three part time jobs and take a full course load. I make the Dean's List every semester so I can maintain good standing with my scholarship requirements. I graduate in four years because that is the length of time my scholarship is available to me. I am a first-generation college student. I walk to the Dollar Store with a trash bag in tow to do my shopping. This is where I get my cereal, canned goods, cleaning spray, toothpaste.

When I move in with my boyfriend a few years later, I hear a roommate and his girlfriend laughing hysterically exiting the bathroom. Other roommates at various times have welcomed their partners to live with them, unofficially and without paying more rent. I am working a full-time job as an assistant manager, and as a barista part-time. I go days without seeing the sun. I am always at work. I pay rent for a shared room. I contribute universal toiletries.

Recently, I put a bottle of free soap from my dad in the main bathroom.

"Did you read that soap bottle?" the roommate's girlfriend asks, still cackling. "It's perineal cleaner!"

She is shrieking now.

"That's for your butt!"

My dad sold our restaurant when I was in middle school, his first retirement, if you can call it a retirement while still being a self-employed business owner, landlord, and part-time custodian at the local hospital. His first day? They make him clean up the afterbirth in a delivery room.

He's supposed to throw away the partially used toiletries in the hospital room once a patient's left. Germs, I guess.

He doesn't. He's been secretly bringing them home. My parents' home, my sister's, and mine are stocked with half empty Kleenex boxes and pump bottles of hospital soap, which is, apparently, perineal cleaner. We've all been using it on our hands.

I look at the lotion he gave me. It says it's good for diaper rash.

My Grandma Marion was a child during the cholera epidemic. Families were told to burn blankets, clothes, and toys. Anything that could carry disease.

Her father was walking by a trash can one day and spotted a beautiful doll inside. One of the Dionne quintuplets, media stars and sensations of their time. He is not supposed to touch it.

The doll is meant to be burned. Instead, my great-grandfather took the doll home to his daughter, my Grandma Marion. Widowed and fallen on perpetual hard times, he weighed the risks, and sought to offer a gift to a child with so little. He had nothing else to give.

* * *

Since graduation I've lived paycheck to paycheck, most of the time with at least two jobs, despite one being full-time. I make decisions from a place of worry and anxiety, but still hope for the best.

I'm married, but we don't have children because we can't afford them. We travel when we can. I wanted to get my finances in order. I went to a financial planner once, but he kept unfolding and folding a graph in front of me that I did not understand, so when I got home, I cried.

Despite him, and others, I managed to get debt free this year. I still find myself panicking more days than not. But when my friends ask for my help or suffer a loss, I give. And I give generously. Because I know what it feels like to grieve, to be looked down on, to need help, to lack.

My father has retired for the third time this year. Maybe this one will stick. Who knows?

He still wears mostly t-shirts he earned from walkathons in the 90s, a longtime Relay for Life participant. He's been a community donor for forever in some capacity or another – cakes for fundraisers, blood drives for the hospital, so much to the church.

He's actually angered my mother he gives so much away. They live paycheck to paycheck, too.

But when I go home to visit, I always wind up finding a couple bills of cash squirreled away in a coat pocket or thrown into my glove box when I get back. A thank you from my dad. He knows if he tries to give it to us in person, we won't accept it. A prideful trait we've learned, in fact, from him.

My grandmother has passed now. As a kid, my strongest memory of her is from family dinners at my parents' restaurant. Filling up a long table with aunts and uncles and cousins, we'd be some of the last to eat again, planning a time when Dad could step away from the kitchen to join us.

Grace would be said, but before the adults could head up to the buffet line, my Grandma Marion would send all the grandkids up to the sweets table for dessert first. This was our tradition.

"To make sure you have room."

Like her father for her, like mine for me, she wanted better for us with what little she could offer.

***

I inherited my hard work ethic from my father, as he learned from his parents. But I also inherited anxiety and periods of depression from living so long in a state of survival. When you operate much of your life from a position of scarcity, even good times feel like they need a contingency plan. Like you better play Orphan again. Because you know it can always get worse. It can always be hard again.

My family is full of people who do what they need to get by. We work the jobs no one else wants. We work multiple jobs because one doesn't pay all the bills. We reuse things, sometimes stealing them when we're not supposed to, because we see purpose and functionality and caring where others see waste. We don't ask for help very often, and because of that, we don't often seek mental healthcare when we need it.

They say money doesn't buy you happiness, but it does buy you peace of mind. It does buy you opportunities. It does buy you time. From generation to generation, we each try to do a little more, a little better than the ones who came before us, not out of disrespect or ingratitude. But because it's what we know they would want for us. What they would give to us willingly if they could.

I know that the way I was raised and the stories I was brought up on have shaped me to be a diligent, passionate, purpose-driven person. I am proud of my family. We are empathizers because we know struggle so intimately. Yet, I also know that scarcity mindset has plagued my opinion of money in general, and my self-esteem. I assume those with money must not be working as hard as me or must have achieved their success through entitlements I don't carry, which, if we're being honest is true in our country, more often than not. Still, I have a constant need for recognition of my work from outsiders. I have the unhealthy habit of comparing myself to others or finding myself in a position where I know they are judging me and placing me lower on their ladder because of the soap in my bathroom or because I eat dessert for breakfast instead of something more sensible. I must be broke ass. I must be nonsensical.

As much as their comments and stares upset me, the worst opinions come from myself. I'm the first person to tell myself I'm not measuring up. I need to work harder. I need to get more done. I need to stop talking to myself so negatively, but that would be easier if I wasn't so disappointing all the time.

The truth is my family, like so many other families, has been sold the idea of the American Dream. We believed working hard would lead to success, but what if working hard really just led us to being tired all the time and stealing half used bottles of butt soap?

I think about the promise for a better life. A life where I'm not worrying about money and how to make ends meet. The moments that must have come up in my Grandma Marion's and my father's life too. I think about the American Dream and how it's a lot closer to that one roommate of mine who stole all my dishes, put them in a see-through bin, and told me *she* never used them.

Perhaps the biggest truth is that I'm afraid I will live a life where I just keep working and working and never hit the made-up line of success regardless. Someone else is making the money. Someone else is taking the credit. Someone else is going to replace me after I'm gone. I will die and be forgotten.

I understand these biases and behaviors are coping mechanisms. I shouldn't be so hard on myself for doing what I needed to do to get by. I have come a long way. I managed to get debt free despite, or maybe out of spite – *who can tell*, when others made me feel small for not understanding a graph or a word I never learned before. I did the best I could with what I knew. Now, I recognize that at various points in my day, and my life, I am my grandmother feeling unwanted. I am my father with stories no one knows. I am still playing the game Orphan.

I don't know how to ask for help very well yet. While never outrightly spoken by my family, to admit I struggle with depression feels like it'd be another failure. In my eyes more than theirs. We work hard! We don't need help! It's tough to shake some stories, even when you know listening to them is a disservice to yourself. So, I carry on, showing up to work, ignoring the toxic environment around me, as well as the one going on in my own head. I take ibuprofen like it's the antidepressants I need but can't afford. On the upside though, I still have hope.

At various points in my day, and my life, I am a doll plucked from the trash and gifted out of pure, maybe ignorant, love. But that's a big amount of love. I am two twenty-dollar bills that fall out of the glove box two weeks after I was left there, showing up just when you need it. That's a saving grace. I am a person you can call on your worst day and I'll listen and help how I can and give even when I don't have a lot. That's a friendship.

I inherited my hard work ethic from my family. I inherited my mental health issues too. People who know me say I have a hard time letting things go, and they're right. My baggage is full of pride and shame, of perseverance and insecurity. It's full of half used boxes of Kleenex because who wouldn't need a tissue after hearing a story like this? What I must remember is that I'm not carrying this baggage alone. I am not, as I feared, an orphan. I am one member of a family who works hard at work, but who also works hard at loving one another. Sometimes we just need to do a better job of loving ourselves.

Bio: Jess Witkins is a Wisconsin-based writer, freelancer, and storyteller. Her work has been published in local and national magazines. She is president of the nonprofit writing community, Mississippi Valley Writers Guild. Most recently her poems have appeared in *Ariel Chart* and *Rising Phoenix Review.* She has an essay titled "The Funeral Photographer" in the anthology, *What Remains: The Many Ways We Say Goodbye,* with Gelles Cole Literary Enterprises.

WITHIN AND WITHOUT SKIN

by Dominica Selvaggio

The first time I heard my "father's" name was when I visited my birth mother, Diane, in a hospital bed. She was surrounded by equipment to help her COPD ridden lungs keep oxygen cycling after a lifetime of smoking. But, by some grace, she had enough breath to tell me a story. I was 23 years old. It was only my second time meeting my mother as an adult since I had been separated from her as a child at the age of four. The age of foster care.

Fire burned through me as I listened to the tale she wove of my beginnings –something never told to me.

Diane and Nick met because he owned a club in the Southside of Chicago, in the Cicero neighborhood. My mother was working as a sex worker at the time. A trade inherited from her mother, an exotic dancer at the age of sixteen.

Diane said that my father was Charming. Powerful. Cunning. *Brown.*

I tried to ask questions. My mouth wouldn't speak, and Diane wouldn't offer any other information. She made me promise to not go looking for him. Convinced that he would ask me to get involved in trafficking drugs – something she said he had done to his other children.

Maybe that's true. Or maybe my mother was racist.

She seemed desperate in telling me to stay away from him. All I could hear was my father's blood pounding in my ears. Echoes of rage.

There's no way of asking her any more details because she died from the flame a mere four years after this sterile room conversation. And so, I clung to the story of my white-passing biracial identity until a DNA test shattered that "reality".

An origin story eliminated.

The only bit of my father erased.

A connection to LatinX culture – *false.*

I am more colonizer than anything else.

What is an identity, if not a story?

In my experiences as a 31-year-old, late life foster kid/ adoptee, complex childhood sexual trauma survivor, queer, trans/non-binary human, and Licensed Mental Health Counselor with a long list of disabilities/mental health conditions, I have come to realize that healing doesn't only come from having an integrated sense of self and safety in identity – it comes when we can see the places in which we intersect. When we can trust the ways in which we are connected and held.

A bridge cannot connect lands without stretching over divides.

How do you join darkness and light?

Through being forced to reckon with my own ambiguous racial identity story, internalized racism, the shame/ fragility/complicity/violence that comes with whiteness, and both receiving/providing clinical care in the privatized mental health care system, I am deeply invested in the questions –

How can a person cultivate mental wellness when the system is designed for them to feel unwell?

How does a person access safety when the monster is perceived both within and without the skin?

I decided to ask those whose stories offer a clearer and more precise perspective than mine alone can offer, fully realizing that my pen is also influenced by whiteness – which is why you won't find my words in the essay below.

What you are about to read is a story that has been woven from interviews with three extraordinary BIPOC (Black, Indigenous, and people of color) people about their experiences with race and mental health/healing. Each person was first given an outline of what the interview/essay would be about, compensated for their time/emotional labor, and given full editing rights to the narrative being told.

Quotes from each persons' interview have been pulled and braided to form a larger story.

Threads are stronger when woven together. They create new worlds.

•

G = Gabes Torres (she/they), a Filipnx woman of color who is currently based in Duwamish territory- widely known as Seattle, WA. She is a psychotherapist, researcher, artist, and speaker who does antiracism and decolonizing work in the realms of mental health, education, and creativity.

V = Val (she/her), a Black Seattle based spiritual wellness practitioner dedicated to her own healing journey as well as holding space for others on theirs.

B = Britt Wilson (she/her), a Black Breathwork facilitator, healing justice advocate who is healing herself and her community.

•

G: I know who I am, and I know what my yeses and nos are. *It was a costly journey to be able to be at this place.*

Being born and raised in the Philippines, being raised in a Filipino and Christian context, the conversations around themes in mental health and emotions and feelings of disappointment are not as welcome.

V: I wasn't taught to talk about my feelings, so I rarely did. There was this fear of being othered. The fear of hearing people talk about it and me. I held everything inside always.

G: There is a massive hesitation amongst BIPOC, especially Black folks, especially Black men who choose not to pursue therapy because of being susceptible to being pathologized.

Rage being pathologized. Grief being pathologized.

B: My father – my biological father – suffered a lot with his mental health and addiction and I don't think that was ever fully addressed while he was alive. That's something I think about often.

The first time I remember going to therapy was like in the fourth or fifth grade, and that my first therapist was actually a Black therapist. I have had issues with depression and anxiety and suicidality, and I was hospitalized when I was in eighth grade for attempted suicide.

V: My very first experience with mental health was right around the time of my parent's divorce. I went to a therapist because my dad found out that I was cutting. I wasn't suicidal, but I was self-harming as a way of getting attention from my parents.

To make them see me.

G: Symptomatology is important. You should be able to see the manifestations of trauma and of *dis-ease.* Not disease.

There is this continuous narrative around Black and brown minds and Black and brown people being the subjects of study/experimentation in non-consensual ways. Which is again a narrative of colonialism, because non-consensual is invasive and it involves subjugation. It is unwelcomed.

V: Growing up, mental health wasn't something that was talked about within the Black community at all. Especially not within my family. My parents are from Haiti – which is a different layer. People in Haiti will say, "Oh, that person is depressed," but not really know what to do with it. Or they'll be like, "Pray."

It does get to be a lot to take, and I feel like a lot of other Black people can relate to that. We even talk about the trope of the "strong Black woman." Do you know how many Black women die in childbirth alone – not just in childbirth – but throughout any routine medical procedure, because people see us as so "strong"?

We are still human.

B: When I started going to middle school and I was the only Black kid in a very white wealthy area – that was one thing, then I was hospitalized right after that. In high school, I was on medication almost the entire time. In college, I was coming up for air because I was off medication and I was in a different environment. Things had been going relatively well, but there was this low grade *dis-ease.*

G: BIPOC end up generally being defined as "abnormal." White is regarded as the standard – and everything else is "diverse."

That's what ends up happening with the lack of representation in the Mental Health and Psychology fields. Just because a Black or brown immigrant of color, or migrant of color, just so happens to relate and engage and exist in ways that are different, doesn't mean that they are defective. And for the longest time that has been the narrative.

That we are unwell.

It goes back to education. It goes back to the access to the education in the first place. And who's writing the textbook and who's educating. It's always going to be a politicized process.

Wellness is political. Pleasure is political.

V: We have to fit ourselves into these molds just to be accepted and, even then, we are not fully accepted. You tell us to play by your rules and we do. We jump through all of the hoops – just to continue to be paid less, or to be passed up for promotions, or to be passed up for different opportunities, and so on.

My mental health just tanked. There was nothing wrong with my life, I was going on autopilot and going through the motions. I tried finding a Black therapist, and that is something that is super hard in Seattle. I couldn't find it.

G: In order to survive and be protected, we have to disassociate from the varied tones that elicit threat or stimulate white bodies. We cannot erase the melanin from our skin.

B: Obviously I walk around in a Black body, and so going out into the world and seeing police officers is definitely a trigger.

At the same time, because nothing has happened to me personally, I disassociate. I think it's a trauma response. It's like, "I'm not in this body- they don't see me – nothing will happen." At the same time, I have to remind myself that "you are in this body – you are here right now – this is a very real thing that happens."

V: I just remember when we found out about Ahmaud Arbery, and it was like, "Fuck, this is happening again." It still is almost disassociated for me. It didn't hit me until George Floyd died.

We didn't even get to really go through this.

I remember having a complete breakdown. I had to take time off work, because right after that the protesting started.

I've been to two protests because I've been really nervous about them and not knowing what could happen to me.

B: Let all those white people go out there and protest. I'm going to be here and enjoy my body. Because I think for generations, we, especially as Black women, have learned to shoulder and carry the weight for everyone else and what I'm tapping into is that need for *radical rest.*

G: The fact that race is a construct – a social construct that also has a visual component to it. It's not a form of oppression Olympics. It's a way of seeing how people live in many different worlds because of how they are perceived and treated by the world.

And if it is a race then there are some people who start at a later time of the race or who don't even have shoes to begin with.

V: Trauma is held in the body. It starts off in the mind, and then seeps through, and becomes those physical representations. You can't heal from it if you're not aware of it.

You can't heal it if you don't feel it.

B: We are all born into these systems of white supremacy and anti-Blackness, and we all have to take those steps to unlearning. It is impossible not to internalize.

It is literally in the air we breathe.

G: And for those who are not white – they are regarded – even if it wasn't intended or it was implicitly on unconsciously done – as sub-human. And what has always been the core of white supremacy is that there is this internalized hierarchy of human dignity, and at the very top are white people. Are whiteness. Are straightness. Ability. It just goes on.

And there is a representation of this gnostic tradition around the flesh – or bodies – being bad. And that things that are transcendent or of god are morally good.

B: I had a ton of internalized racism growing up in white spaces. Right before I moved to Seattle, I experienced one of the deepest depressions I have ever had in my life. I was going through one of those chapters where I was like, "I don't want to be here anymore." That feeling of being trapped and being *a victim to your own mental circumstances.*

I have to remind myself – it's literally not real.

G: It is a survival mechanism to disconnect, and a lot of cultures that are non-western or non-white are the most embodied. We are more in touch with our movement. It's where yoga originated, and where mindfulness/meditation originated. If we look into Black and brown churches, they are more synced with their rhythm and their bodily swaying.

B: After that I found a Black therapist, who is the best therapist I've ever had in my life, I started practicing breathwork. I think it was the combination of having the support from her and having the breath work that gave me the most healing that I've experienced in a mental health setting.

V: My first-time experiencing Reiki, I remember lying down, closing my eyes, and it being so cool to be able to feel my energy. I was holding onto a lot at the time. It felt like she pulled something huge out of my chest.

B: It brought some intactness, like some pieces came together.

G: Every person has a different journey or path to healing because of their identity. *A Western approach of mental health looks at the symptom – whereas a decolonized one looks at the story.*

I know that I have very little access to my ancestors, precolonial time. I found out recently that I'm second generation first nation's Filipino. They're called the Aeta.

I have been leaning into the wisdom and guidance of my ancestors. I would lean into our history – not just our intergenerational trauma and pain and struggle and resistance – but also our medicine, our resilience, and *celebrating who we are as us.*

V: I found my way to this beautiful healing program that really changed my life. That was my first taste of what it feels like to be in community. And spiritual community. Where I could be vulnerable. *We could cry together.*

G: The idea that I'm a part of a collective or an ecological reality is my starting point. I am my own, and also, I am of a community.

Who are you in this world? What are the intersecting identities that make you, "you?" And how then do you practice anti-racism? Especially if you have racial and class privilege and ability privilege and cis privilege and all the privileges – I would then ask you – not if you are racist but how you are racist.

B: That's something that has been missing for a big bulk of my healing journey. I needed to be amongst other people and share that healing. I'm learning every single day how to be in community – which is the opposite of white supremacy.

G: We talk about white supremacy and racism and the varied factors and individuals who continue to oppress us. We talk a lot about what we could be free from.

But what can we be free for?

B: I'm becoming more familiar and intimate with joy and what that feels like. For me, it has felt like laughing out loud at something on tv, or being present with friends, or getting a good workout in.

But at the same time – when I feel that sense of guilt coming up – I tell myself, "Haven't you lived a lifetime of this? Isn't it ok for you to be ok with not having to worry about that for a little bit?"

G: This is why joy as a revolution and pleasure as a revolution are significant – it's because we are finally talking about who we are, what we are about, who we are about, and us just being us – and part of precolonial or decolonial experiences is that it was just us being us, untouched and uninvaded, if such a word exists, by the colonizer.

V: My sense of power comes when I am being my *most authentic self.* I'm not so fixated on trying to be perfect for anyone else or trying to get their validation. I just give myself permission to be myself and to love on myself.

G: Being hospitable to my ancestors is joyful. Because consent and invitation are not things that they experienced because of the history of colonialism, and, for me, the way that I caress, and care, and protect my skin, my face, my body – how I take my time, and how I sing and speak in my language – and that being a revolution because *I am no longer ashamed of my flesh.*

V: If your power is fueled by joy and gratitude, it hits differently because it's clean energy. You're not taking from someone. You're not harming anyone else.

G: Racism is both a behavioral and a systemic reality that everybody is not without prejudice. It just so happens that there are people who have the institutional power to carry out their prejudice.

B: Resources would be great. Resources and having access to Black practitioners, healers, therapists, social workers, doctors, and people who look like us in these spaces.

How would my father's life have been different had he had access to the resources he needed?

G: That is why Black and Indigenous folks cannot be racist, because they do not have the institutional power to be able to carry out prejudice. So, there's no such thing as reverse racism.

V: We are human, and we are vulnerable. We are not permanent here. *Our bodies aren't permanent here.*

G: No matter how much monetary benefit that QTBI-POC communities have – money is not going to be the thing that undoes our centuries of intergenerational trauma, but it helps build systems that will.

B: Holding breathwork space for more BIPOC people is healing that part of me, too, as someone who struggled with their identity for a really long time. There's only so much healing you can do by yourself. We are social creatures – we need each other – we need to see ourselves reflected in each other.

V: Whenever I'm able to hold space for other people's healing, it's a connected mutual feeling of power. When I'm able to uplift other people, it brings me so much joy.

G: There's a South African philosophy – it's Ubuntu. *I am because we are.*

B: There's so many great practitioners and healers out there creating spaces and putting themselves at the fore-front and it's so lovely to see that. I'm thinking of the pictures I've seen on Instagram of communities of Black women in spaces together healing. That's what I want.

V: I am really happy that so many more Black people are looking at mental health, at the trauma, at why we have the anger that we hold, and at the sadness that we hold.

B: Honestly, being Black is being in the best club ever! It's so comforting to know that so many of us have had that same experience and to have that level of intimacy and understanding with each other. No matter what bull-shit is going on in the world, we always find ways to laugh and find humor and be funny.

G: The antidote to the thing is not the thing itself. *We are finding healing and redemption within us.*

•

These were not easy conversations. Bravery, boundaries, compassion, laughter, and grounding were required. These humans' courage, resilience, healing practices, languages, and stories are gifts that are not owed.

I am grateful. So grateful.

I started writing as a way to heal myself. To find my voice. To reclaim my story. To write myself into existence. Now I write myself into relationship – an ambiguous place with more questions than answers that's often fraught with conflict and heart.

And so, I ask myself and I ask us all –

How can we create communities in which it is safe to be vulnerable?

How can we take the armor off? Is it safe to do so?

When is the last time you truly listened to someone who is different than you?

How can we repair the harm that has been caused?

What is justice?

What is forgiveness?

What is accountability?

What if all flesh was rejoiced?

I would like to thank Gabes, Britt, and Val once again for sharing their hearts and for trusting me to tell their stories.

I would like to acknowledge and thank the land (widely known as Portland) of the Multnomah, Wasco, Cowlitz, Kathlamet, Clackamas, Bands of Chinook, Tualatin, Kalapuya, and Molalla tribes for the residence that supported this project.

And I would like to thank you, dear reader, for making it this far.

Because we have a long way to go before the tapestry is whole.

Bio: Within and Without Skin is a braided essay that explores the intersections of race and the mental health care system, written by the adoptee, queer/non-binary writer, Dominica Selvaggio (they/them). Dominica is a white bodied Licensed Mental Health Counselor deeply invested in dismantling the systems of white-bodied supremacy, colonialism, patriarchy, ableism, heteronormativity, and capitalism, as these systems are largely responsible for the negative mental health outcomes for marginalized folks. You can find more of their work in the pages of Papeachu Press, For Women Who Roar, This is Jane Project, Wussy Magazine, and Project Heal.

BETTER TO TRAVEL HOPEFULLY THAN TO ARRIVE

by Essam Sannoufi

Translated by Gillian Oliver

BLACKPOOL, UK, 2017

The letter bore the stamp of the UK health service and had all the warmth of a legal judgement. Dear Essam, it started, though it was not personally signed.

It reminded me that I had recently been assessed by a mental health charity for stress relating to physical health, and no further action was required. They didn't wish to hear from me again and had closed my case.

I felt strangely elated that I was not considered either mentally unstable or open to radicalization, but downcast because my constant sense of isolation was not recognized. How I longed for the safety of Syria, and all the love that was there for me.

HOMS, SYRIA, 2013

The impact was like an electric shock. It delivered me face down on the road. My stomach had been hit and I knew it.

But I could wiggle my toes, so I hoped the damage wasn't that bad.

By instinct my friends started running towards me, but I begged them to stay back. We all knew how snipers worked, here in Old Homs. From their hidden vantage points they would be watching for the ones who came to my aid, ready to strike again.

HOMS, 2010

Like me, all my friends came from families that went back generations in the city of Homs. The oldest Christian church in the world was there, tucked in among all the mosques. My best friends were Christian and there wasn't a trace of racism in my boyhood world.

We weren't rich, but we had everything: sunshine and sea, watermelons and bulgur wheat, petrol and gas, families and a future. And though my brothers joined my father in the family greengrocer's, I had other plans. I was studying French literature and started a graphic design business.

Yes, it was heavenly. But I think you would always want to stay in the place you grew up, even if it was just three trees on a road.

Homs became famous when it was destroyed in the war, but it's been under threat of attack for generations. The big, old city gates stood for centuries against the marauding hordes that wanted to dominate us.

Legend has it that Homs was once saved not by might, but by guile.

Once, when Mogul forces arrived in anger, they were surprised to find residents tearing their clothes and talking nonsense. The invaders assumed the water was poisoned and departed. That's when 100,000 people dropped their act and celebrated being saved from the sword. Today, if you ask anyone in Syria, they'll say, "Oh, in Homs, they're all crazy," and they will laugh.

The joke is on the one who underestimates the Homsi people.

HOMS, 2013

I tried to pull myself forward using my hands and arms, but something was pulling me back. I looked over my shoulder and saw my leg broken, sprawling at an angle with the bone exposed. The pain was immense, and the weight of my broken leg held me in place on my stomach in the road.

There were no ambulances or hospitals, but somehow, I found myself first in a car and then in a shallow underground bunker staffed with volunteer medics. I slept for ten hours under the anesthetic they gave me.

After about twelve hours, we all wondered why my catheter bag was devoid of urine. The doctors said, "Why don't you try to pee, Essam, and we'll see what happens."

Turns out, the sniper's bullet had entered my left hip and exited on my right, searing the tube from my bladder out of my body. When I pushed, my urine breached the obstruction and ran into my abdomen, which lay cut and bleeding inside.

Do you know if you have a tiny nick on your finger and you get alcohol on it, how much it smarts? Imagine that pain whooshing through your sliced internal organs. It was excruciating.

In that bunker I had time to consider my new state: 24 years old and disabled. I had prepared for only two options – being victorious or being dead.

HOMS, 2013

No one was expecting a President Assad.

When you open a book in Syria, or go anywhere from a launderette to petrol station, you see the picture of Assad's father, Hafez al-Assad and his eldest son and heir, Bassel

– Bassel in a plane, riding a horse, or standing on top of a hill. Bassel was the one they were preparing for power.

But when Bassel died in "an accident," his younger brother Assad was next in line.

When I say, "in line," please do not think Syria is a kingdom with a royal family. It is nominally a republic. In fact, it is a dictatorship.

Assad was too young to be president; he was only 34. You need to be over 40 to be president of Syria. It took the parliament about five minutes to change the law in Assad's favor. No one argued about it; that wasn't allowed.

And no one really knew much about Assad. People said, "He looks kind. He is a doctor. He probably wants to change things. It will take ages."

Those who had lived through the events of 1982 said little. They recalled how Assad's father slaughtered 40,000 Syrians in three weeks and destroyed their city. In those days, the militia would murder you in the street without cause. Perhaps this new, young president would be better, but he could be even worse.

But my generation came after 1982. We had mobile phones and social media. We were open minded, with a strong feeling about freedom. We were willing to stand up and speak out.

And that's how I, a university student and a graphic designer, became part of the resistance. I created campaigns, banners, and posters. These asked where the food and fuel had gone, why there was no medicine for the children. I was hopeful of emboldening others.

And on that day, laden with boxes of handbills, I crossed the road I always crossed.

There was a barricade set up across it, to protect those in the resistance from snipers. It was sagging a bit in the middle that day. I looked over the top of it as I crossed.

Was it my fault I was hit? I put my head above the parapet.

HOMS, 2013

"Essam needs to get out of here." The good doctors of the bunker could only help you stay alive, not get better. They tried to find a legal way to move me on for further treatment, but it didn't work.

I had my friends around me. They sat by my side day and night and took care of my most basic physical needs. They made their way around the broken open houses of Old Homs looking for bulgur or dried fruit and medicines, garnering supplies for me.

And in the end, as we judged there was no other option, they carried me out on their shoulders. The journey to Lebanon from Old Homs takes five minutes by road, but four hours by foot and in the shadows, as we had to escape in secret. It was a route with deep trenches, through woods with flooded fields and rivers. At some points in the journey, my friends were in over their heads.

I was just lying on a stretcher, but it took as much energy as running. I was so worried that something would happen to my friends.

They had loved and supported me from their hearts. Three of them delivered me to the safe region and then returned to Old Homs. All three died in a siege after returning. Later, I would recall the gift of their company compared to the bleakness of travelling alone.

New friends began the dealmaking to get me to Lebanon. Money must have changed hands because, after a week of waiting, we were told, "There is a route; get ready." I went by motorbike and taxi – the journey took one full day.

On the borders of Lebanon, the Red Cross had built a base to support injured Syrians. The doctors there were upbeat. They smiled, and I caught their confidence. I really thought that, in three months, I'd be back on my feet. After all, they had things like an MRI scanner – such things had been destroyed in Syria's war.

But dark clouds gathered as the truth of my situation emerged. Lebanon would not be a six-month stopover on the way to full recovery. The happy doctors could fix my broken leg, but their interventions to fix my ruptured internal organs had created more problems. My injuries required a type of rare specialist that was not easy to find.

I disappeared into depression when it turned out my hopes were in vain. I sunk into a three-day void, during which time I fully desired to be like my friends who died. I saw them as very lucky, to be admired, as if they had just graduated from university to become doctors.

In this darkness, and in this pain, I became like a person outside of myself – even with someone advocating for me, pressing my case. I hear him say, "I understand why Essam is sad. He has no options at the moment, but he has never stopped trying to do the right thing."

LEBANON, SEPTEMBER 2016

Great Britain has a rich imperial history. It's one of the wealthiest countries in the world. Its health service is advanced like Switzerland or Canada; the world's best doctors live there.

London and Birmingham had surgeons who knew about war wounds, but the United Kingdom's Home Office did not send me to London or Birmingham.

Instead, I was on a flight to Manchester, buoyed by the sense of a new beginning and the smiles and warmth of the crew. On touchdown, well-wishers greeted us from all corners of the county. We were smoothly bussed to a children's center, where the local mosque had laid on a spread fit for heroes. "Welcome to the most beautiful town in England," said the Imam with wide open arms.

After three years without official papers, this was a gift greater than any of us could recall. I could finally see a way to my operation, and then to my future, a marriage and a family, and a way to earn a living.

But the UK government instead sent me from Manchester to the poorest local authority in England, Blackpool, far away from the surgeons I needed. Without money or status, I was wholly in the hands of the local government integration team. While I had rights relating to their resettlement program, asserting those rights would not be easy. In fact, it would get me into trouble, and I knew it.

"You can walk fine, I see," said the integration manager, setting the tone for our future encounters.

BLACKPOOL, JANUARY 2017

Not being believed about my injuries was not part of my experience in Syria or Lebanon, but it became one of the most enduring and bewildering aspects of being in Britain.

I carried medical records from the United Nations spelling out the nature of my injuries and subsequent complications from surgery.

From my own understanding of these, I had hoped to be transferred from the airport to the operating table upon arrival.

But notwithstanding my rudimentary English, it was my job to arrange my treatment. And despite knowing the operation couldn't happen at the local hospital, I had to begin there, and work my way up to the more distant surgeons I knew I needed.

Four months after I arrived in the UK, I achieved my first appointment. At Blackpool's hospital, the uncertain doctor wavered. "Which should come first, this operation or that one?" he asked me. He wanted to send a camera down to investigate – an endoscopic procedure. I begged: "Oh, please, spare me that pain! I know it from before and it takes me days to recover."

He relented, saying, "You need to try Manchester. I can't help you here."

MANCHESTER, OCTOBER 2017

A journey by train to a hospital in Manchester felt like a trip to the moon. This concerned the most important aspect of my life, after all. I could not possibly be late for the appointment or be unable to pay for it. The integration manager told me the cost of the hospital appointment was included, but they could neither pay for the train ticket there or back, nor accompany me.

The national government advises councils to pay for transport for refugees up to 50 miles. As Manchester is 51 miles from Blackpool, the council declined to pay for my ticket. When I pointed out I had been placed in Blackpool, and this was not my personal choice, the decision went up the council's chain of command.

After these discussions they relented, but I now know they noted me as difficult: "Essam is asking for things."

At my appointment in Manchester, the surgeon had some news of her own. She was about to have a baby, and I would have to wait nine more months for my operation. She said it as if nine months was the same as one week! Even one month felt like a hundred to me.

Twelve months on from my arrival in Britain, clarity came. There was no other surgeon in Manchester able to undertake my treatment. The only place this could happen was in Birmingham or London.

Alone on the train journey home, I reflected. Like the moments after the shooting, I felt I was trying to pull myself forwards while being pulled backwards.

BLACKPOOL, 2017

"Now do you believe me?"" I blurted out to the council officers. "What more do you need from me to show I do need a specialist? I need this treatment for my life to begin."

"So now, take my UN records; ask them to find me treatment anywhere else in the world – I am declaring to you now I will go wherever it is, and I can leave tomorrow."

Their faces indicated that they had never heard anything like it. An internal council memo recorded, "Essam is angry. Essam is shouting."

My transfer request was declined and the business of asking for a train ticket started all over again.

A return ticket to Birmingham from Blackpool costs over £100; I had about half of that.

Yet they would not pay for the ticket and treated me as if I was asking for money to go sightseeing.

Even if I hated someone, I would still try to support them if they had a problem with their health. The 'integration team' of the local council (or government) had one job. It was to stop me from feeling lonely. It was to fight any sense of isolation. In this, they failed.

It wasn't the council staff who visited me twice a week who hated me. One even offered to go to Birmingham with me, but her request was denied. This confirmed it; somewhere in the system, someone hated me. Maybe not only me, maybe all Syrians.

I got to thinking, "I'd like them to like me, but if they don't, I don't care. I need an operation near where I live, or some way to get me there."

There is a government program which looks out for people who could tip into terrorism. These will be angry people. When it was suggested to me in this context that I should have my mental health assessed, I was not surprised. I had prepared myself.

It was another way for them to exercise their power over me. It was their way of threatening me, of keeping me quiet. While this question mark was over me, they could prevent me from working.

I agreed to go ahead with their allegation that I was becoming radicalized before their eyes. I would cooperate with their mental health assessment, though I saw it as a distraction from the treatment I desperately needed.

BLACKPOOL, FEBRUARY 2018

I finally received notice of an operation with a date and a time. This came almost two years after my arrival in Britain. I would have to arrive at the hospital in Birmingham by 7 am on the day of the operation.

At the council's offices, I put a piece of paper on the desk detailing every step of my upcoming journey. I make sure I list every aspect, so they don't have the opportunity to say, "I don't see why this or that is necessary." And it is clear: there simply isn't an option that gets me there by train if I travel on the day of the operation.

And how I would come back afterwards? I didn't know. I wrote down the details: This operation is between my legs, and I will be walking with a bag, a catheter. It may be that they take a slice out of the inside of my cheek to create the missing flesh they need. This will be difficult. I will be in the hospital for three days after the surgery. I will have emptied my stomach and will not have eaten for hours.

They followed all this. They agreed to pay my train fare and for a hotel room the night before the operation. This is the main deal, after all, this is the operation.

But they refused to pay for anyone to accompany me.

BIRMINGHAM, JUNE, 2018

Because I was afraid, I didn't sleep well. Usually I am stronger, but I knew the details of what was about to happen. It was a bad night. It was the most important day I'd been waiting for.

I knew the nurses would prepare me, that I would change my clothes an hour before the surgery, that I would be greeted by the smells and sounds of the hospital. When I remember it now, I feel dizzy.

But this was my reality; there were no other options. I tried to talk with the nurses just as they put in the injection, and I remember the last second before sleeping.

When I woke up after 24 hours, I didn't remember any English words – not even "hi". This was the effect of the anesthetic – this lasted one hour.

After the surgery they monitored me, and on the third day they said, "Today's the day you'll be discharged, around 6 pm."

I said, "Oh, please, I am going home by train; I need three or four hours. Can I please go earlier or later?"

They were incredulous that I was to make the journey by train, but they couldn't do anything to help me. I'm sure it was too far to help me with an ambulance.

Changing trains, I felt I would fall over. My face was very yellow, and I was very slim. I was weak, and I knew it.

BLACKPOOL, JUNE, 2018

The integration officer took one look at me and her eyes flashed wide with realization. She knew at once they had made a big mistake.

"Look, Essam," she said. "For your next appointment we will pay for someone to go with you."

But by now I know the journey by heart. The treatments ahead are less onerous. I have found a way for the hospital to pay for my travel. I will go by myself. I can leave at three in the morning. I'd rather do that than ask them for help.

I just said, "I am going to make a formal complaint. Please tell me how to do this."

BLACKPOOL, 2019

The ombudsman ruled the council "could have done better," and a minor reshuffle in the council's managerial class followed.

His report offered the thinnest concession that my anger, rather than being a sign of mental instability, was justified. But of the resettlement scheme itself, that it could exasperate even the most moderate person, there was no reflection.

And I could only hope that something might come of the idea that the British state had invested in my isolation more successfully than my integration.

Meanwhile, at a ceremony at the Blackpool Hilton, I was awarded English Student of the Year 2018. I qualified as a community interpreter, got certificates in mathematics and computing, and volunteered with Lancashire Refugee Council.

What trouble that sniper brought with just one bullet. But, from wishing I was dead to asking why I am still alive, I see a light. And the Essam who put his head above the parapet knows what it means:

When I was in such difficulty, I wanted someone to deliver my voice. Now, I want to deliver theirs. There are lots of people with cases like mine.

I am still alive for a big reason, not a small one.

Bio: The revolution of the people of Syria against President Assad began in 2011. In ten years, around half a million people were killed and ten times more escaped the country.

This is Essam Sannoufi's story. He is one of 170,000 refugees permanently resettled out of Syria by the United Nations High Commission for Refugees.

He was in physical pain beyond imagining, though soothed by the love and dedication of friends in Syria. But Essam had to endure another kind of pain: a continuing mental anguish inflicted by state bureaucracy, insensitive to the very person they were supposed to be helping.

THE DAY I BECAME A 'PULLER'

LIVING WITH TRICHOTILLOMANIA

by Chelsea Ohlemiller

Crash.

Windows busted, doors so crunched they cannot be opened. The car is now half the size it once was. There is glass and blood sprinkled over everything. Everyone survived but this scene and experience are brutal. Car rides will never be the same after today. This accident will change who I am forever.

This is the day and moment I became an anxious soul with a messy mind. In a split second my mind shifted to a compulsive, anxious, and fearful place. This wreck and the consequences of the accidental destruction demanded my brain rewire itself. Trauma can do that. Trauma and anxiety are frightful companions.

I slowly find out that anxiety can manipulate your once sound mind into intense compulsions. Compulsions that I can't control. Compulsions that will change my life in more ways than I could imagine. Compulsions that will dictate my future actions and reactions. Compulsions I've never heard of and ones most people around me don't even know exist.

The first time it happens I am lost, confused, and scared. It wasn't an anxiety attack. It was more than that, but I'm just a kid and I don't even know what anxiety is. What I know is that I entered the car with eyes full of thick dark lashes, and I will leave the car with empty eyelids that no one recognizes, including myself.

I had just become a "puller" and someone with trichotillomania, though we won't learn these terms for months to come. I have no clue what this means. I have no concept of what has just happened. I only know that I survived this car ride, even amid paralyzing fear. I arrive at my destination, but I've arrived a different person, both mentally and physically.

The fear of being in a car after the devastating wreck months before caused so much anxiety that I masked the fear with pain and self-mutilation. I didn't consciously choose to pull; it happened. It was my body's response to debilitating and overpowering anxiety and stress. It was a response to trauma.

Who knew that some people's bodies and minds create compulsive pulling as it's "fight or flight" reaction? I wouldn't wish this response on my worst enemy. I didn't know it at the beginning of this diagnosis, but I'll spend the rest of my life wondering why I was cursed with this disorder, this syndrome, and this embarrassing anxiety reaction.

With therapy and new knowledge, we find out the name and the cause of my disorder. My nine-year-old self learns the word *trichotillomania*. My nine-year-old self learns about chemical imbalances in the brain. I learn the acronyms OCD and PTSD. I learn about words like anxiety and stress. I learn more than a kid at my age should know about mental health.

Trichotillomania will change how others look at me. It will change the way I look at myself. It will change my entire life and while I'll do everything I can to make it go away, eventually I'll learn there is no quick fix or cure for this mental health disorder.

Life from here on out is filled with big emotions and big reactions.

If you're like me after a mental health diagnosis, you immediately try to fix and heal. If a solution is offered, you give it an attempt. You try to pray it away. You try to wish it away. You seek therapy. You medicate. You end up zombie-like and still yet to be cured.

The worst part of a mental health diagnosis as a child is that, while you lack a cure at the same time, you also lack the understanding, compassion, and empathy from the kids in your school. You are made fun of, looked at differently, and bullied for the very thing that you'd like to escape from. It's a double-edged sword. You hate and despise the very thing that they do–the way you look, your bald lash line and your sudden transformation. You are just as confused and shocked as those who work tirelessly to humiliate you.

To your peers you have suddenly changed. You're different now. You become a target. Would they make fun of you if they knew your story? Would they make fun of you if they understood the makeup of your brain? Would they make fun of someone with special needs or an incurable disease? Because what you're facing seems like a mixture of both.

Eventually, you find ways to hide the pulling and the way you're unlike everyone else. It isn't a cure but a mask for the battles you face. Eventually, you find ways to prolong the attacks and episodes. Eventually, you find ways to face the world's cruelty toward people who are like you. Eventually, you learn to accept the cyclical timeline of your disorder and learn ways to cope. You don't realize it for a very long time, but you're an overcomer.

With time, you can make the compulsions disappear for long periods of time, until the moment that you can't, and the cycle begins again.

No matter how old you get, the pulling never stops completely – instead, it ebbs and flows with life's encounters. When life is happy, it becomes non-existent. When life is filled with stress or anxiety, it will take over. Pulling has the power to quickly dominate, no matter how long it has been absent.

Into adulthood you will hear peers and colleagues use the phrase, "I'm so stressed I could pull my hair out!", and you'll wonder if these people truly understand the true meaning and creation of that phrase. Deep down you already know the answer: they don't and why would they? Sadly, you do, though you'd desperately wished you didn't. You only know the origin of that expression because you're living it.

One day you find the tools, the strength, and the mind-shift to live with your disorder. Once you learn to live with it, and accept it for what it is, you learn to engage with it differently. That alone makes you a success story.

You are a unique soul living with an anxiety disorder. You are a person living with trichotillomania. More beautifully, you are a person who has the strength, grit, and determination to fight this compulsion and the consequences of it every day. Some days hold success, others hold compulsive episodes, neither hold failure.

There is no complete cure, but you don't need one because you are brave and strong and resilient and you'll live a beautiful life, with or without all of your hair. Even better, maybe there is a cure. Maybe the cure is simply overcoming the shame and embarrassment of living with a trichotillomania label.

For me, there was healing in finally gaining the confidence to feel proud of where I am, to have the vulnerability to share my story with the world so others look at themselves in a different light. One where they aren't alone. One that isn't judged by the sum of their biggest pulling session.

I want little girls, teenagers, adults, and people of all walks of life to read this and realize they are more than this disorder. They are more than the destruction of their mental health struggles. I'm hopeful others struggling with mental illness can stop hiding behind the shame, the embarrassment, and the ridicule and say, "I am more than my flaws. I am more than the sum of my faults. I am more than my anxious mind and fearful thoughts. I am me, and I am beautiful!"

You are beautiful, resilient, and, most of all, you're worthy of a life that isn't defined by your compulsions, anxieties, or fear of diagnosis. You're a mental health warrior, keep charging forward.

Bio: Chelsea Ohlemiller is an educator, speaker, and grief writer who is best known for her authentic portrayal of living life with loss. After the untimely death of her mother, Chelsea created *Happiness, Hope & Harsh Realities*, a blog and social media brand that honors grief and creates a space for others to share in the vulnerable journey of one of life's most universal concepts. Her goal as a writer is to take real-life experiences, both the happy and the harsh, and turn them into something others can relate to. She lives in Indiana with her husband and three children.

HOW TO BE GOOD

by Eden Julia Sugay

Today I thought, *I'd like to treat myself.* I reach for a bag of Good & Gather vegetable straws, which I picked up on my last trip to Target before the first San Francisco Bay Area shelter-in-place went into effect. I turn the bag around to note the suggested serving size and am delighted to see a total of 40 pieces per serving. My usual train of thought leads to some simple math to answer one important question: *If I eat nothing else apart from this entire bag of snacks today, will my total calorie count be less than 1,000?* Turns out, yes! This snack fits that criteria. Instead of eating the suggested serving size of 40 vegetable straws, let alone the entire bag, I pour 20 pieces into a white ceramic bowl and tell myself I am limiting my snacks, trying to make them last longer during these uncertain, challenging times. *I am doing a good thing,* I think. *I am being good.*

Two days earlier, my friends and I drank together during a "Friendship Happy Hour" over Zoom, which has become the new normal. For an inexplicable reason, virtual attention as opposed to in-person fills me with anxiety, so I turn to a complicated coping mechanism: eating. I start snacking on the bottom bits of what was a bag of Baked Hot Cheetos, when one of my friends asks how it's possible I have any left. "Those would be gone by now in my house!" she says. I explain that I'm rationing since we must self-isolate for the foreseeable future, when my other friend adds I had great self-control long before the COVID-19 outbreak. "You're so good," she emphasizes. That's when it dawned on me: Quarantine is allowing me to slip into a pattern of disordered eating again.

For the past 19 months our television screens and timelines have been bursting with news on the COVID-19 pandemic. Between not knowing which news sources to trust, fighting with loved ones on the effectiveness of social distancing, and the current insecurity of our economy putting our lives at risk, it's easy to become lost. It's like every day there is something new to be terrified of. Thankfully, the internet has the capacity to band together to provide much-needed comedic relief, some of which come in the form of memes and challenges on TikTok. Yet not all jokes are harmless. I came across a meme that said, "We are either going to leave this quarantine 50 pounds lighter or 100 pounds heavier," and another similar meme expressing, "The quarantine 15 is the new freshman 15." These memes, born from the pandemic's isolation and delusion of time, create a platform that further highlights our inclination toward fatphobia and the incessant need to police other people's bodies. I wonder, *why are we using what little free time and energy we have to over-obsess about our weight? How can we still be so concerned about what our bodies may look like when people are dying at accelerating rates daily?*

But perhaps we aren't obsessing about weight any more than we normally do; we now just have seemingly endless amounts of time to harshly critique ourselves and falling into that space compounded with the stress of our global state of affairs, is where this isolation can become dangerous for people who experience or are recovering from eating disorders (EDs). The National Association of Anorexia Nervosa and Associated Disorders (ANAD) reports that at least 30 million people in the United States alone suffer from an eating disorder[1]. ANAD also reports that 33-50% of anorexia patients have a comorbid mood disorder, such as depression, though the percentage is much higher in the binge/purge subtype than in the restrictive subtype[2]. I contribute to each of these statistics.

I was diagnosed with bulimia nervosa and binge eating disorder when I was 19, after seeking treatment for my depression a second time. There is hardly a time I can remember where I didn't struggle with food, whether it was eating too much, too little, or not at all, and (to no one's surprise) a great deal of this struggle is a product of my childhood. I didn't have the language to understand or explain body dysmorphia and EDs until later in high school when I secretly saw a counselor behind my parents' backs, but I became exceptionally familiar with the disappointment, frustration, and disgust that accompanied the disorders at a young age.

I am the youngest of five children. My parents immigrated to Southern California from the Philippines in the 70s, with the hopes of providing themselves and their children with better opportunities. They were strict, god-fearing people who placed massive importance on our grades, future professions, and appearances. We had strict computer and phone curfews: computer usage was reserved for homework and needed to be completed by 8 pm, even if we weren't done with our work (not being done with our work meant we were inadequate) and all phones needed to be locked up in our parents' bedroom as soon as we returned from school. Asking for help or advice on

1 "Social Economic Cost of Eating Disorders in US – Harvard University." *Https://Www.hsph.harvard.edu/Striped/Report-Economic-Costs-of-Eating-Disorders/*, Harvard T.H. Chan School of Public Health, June 2020, https://cdn1.sph.harvard.edu/wp-content/uploads/sites/1267/2020/07/Social-Economic-Cost-of-Eating-Disorders-in-US.pdf.

2 Jon Arcelus, LMS. "Mortality Rates in Patients with Anorexia Nervosa and Other Eating Disorders: A Meta-Analysis of 36 Studies." *Archives of General Psychiatry*, JAMA Network, 1 July 2011, https://jamanetwork.com/journals/jamapsychiatry/fullarticle/1107207.

personal matters or trying to approach mental health topics was never encouraged. Asking for help instead represented extreme weakness. I felt very isolated by the constant need to be the best when all other ideas or desires unrelated to academic or professional success were relentlessly silenced. My siblings and I followed this daily routine until we were old enough to leave the house.

My father was an emotional and physical tyrant, while my mother was, at times, a quiet observer intending to mitigate his harm, but other times absent altogether. This thrust me into a deep depression as a child, but I could play the perfect pretender: a happy and content child fulfilled by good grades, a diverse portfolio of talents and hobbies, and an approachable demeanor. Without feeling like I could control much of my own life, I started finding small things I could covertly control, specifically things that related to my body. I started obsessing over my eating patterns when I was 10; a few kids in my class teased me and said no boys would ever like me if I stayed fat. My peers' teasing affected me differently because there were already deep echoes of this insult set into me by my father, who often expressed I wouldn't be able to get a husband if I didn't start taking my body seriously. I was probably 100 pounds at the time. From age 10 to 18 I tried hard to stay around that weight. I would come to find later in life that I accomplished that goal at the expense of my inner peace.

I moved to Northern California in 2010 for college. I fled the constant pressure and surveillance of my home and was finally able to make my own choices. I was trying new things, meeting plenty of wonderful people, and making mistakes and learning from them at my own pace. During my first year of college, I gained weight. You can call it the "freshman 15" or whatever you want, but I started gaining weight because I suddenly felt free to appreciate myself again—I was allowing my body to heal. I entered my second year of college pursuing Creative

Writing and Dance as my majors. Between my second and third years of college, I lost the weight I gained over freshman year, and then I lost some more. A typical day included around three or four dance classes, a few writing seminars and workshops, and an evening workout at the gym. I didn't have time to eat, or maybe I didn't want to give myself the time. I weighed myself every morning as soon as I woke up and every night before I went to bed. I hovered between 93 to 95 pounds those two years and always felt so proud of myself, yet simultaneously so disappointed that I hadn't been able to get below 90. My ED took over once more, with compulsive exercise and anorexia masquerading as a need to stay in shape as a dancer. I would catch myself feeling thrilled by my friends' and family members' praise over my body transformation during this time. I would also feel immediately dissatisfied by the fact I put so much weight on (no pun intended) that thrill.

But it was never enough. I started missing writing workshops and skipping seminars because I was too ashamed of how I looked to leave my room. I watched my hair thin, fall out, and cover every surface of my room. I became too weak to walk to class and some days I didn't get out of bed at all. I spent those days silently tracking the shadows the sun made through my curtains, waiting for the moon to rise so I could attempt sleep. The absences stacked up and my grades suffered. I began risking my scholarships and financial aid, and ultimately my entire enrollment status in college. I was forced to withdraw from courses. I distanced myself further away from others because I didn't want them to see me; I didn't want them to understand how bad everything had become again, I didn't want them to try and help me because I still believed asking for support was wrong and weak, and I didn't want to face the fact that relying on myself wasn't enough. Over this period, I made the difficult decision to stop pursuing my dance studies. I was wrought with guilt, feeling like a quitter, feeling incompetent, feeling like a complete failure who allowed a disorder to win again. I fully dedicated my last year of college to writing but felt small bouts of regret every time I passed rehearsal rooms or ran into my friends from the dance program. It took over three years after graduating in 2014 to finally understand that halting my dance studies meant I *wasn't* allowing my disorder to win again. I have found there are dichotomous misconceptions about what winning and losing both look like. I was raised to believe that needing help in any form was a sign of weakness, that if you resorted to any aid, you've lost. I've been alive for 30 years but have only just begun to appreciate that recognizing your limits doesn't mean your capacities are limited; rather you are acknowledging where you're at and where you can improve, and sometimes being able to improve isn't a solitary journey but one where success can be shared.

***

On top of the quarantine food binge jokes, there are also plenty of jokes about developing alcoholism and increased substance dependence. Sure, I sometimes joke about having a drink during my routine cry-in-the-shower sessions every other day, but the constant barrage of these jokes and images encouraging binge drinking are on a completely different level and are undoubtedly affecting millions of people. Individuals who experience eating disorders often fall into a comorbid addiction. *The Journal of Treatment & Prevention* reported approximately 50% of individuals with an eating disorder either abuse or are dependent on alcohol or illicit substances compared with approximately 9% of the general population[1].

I combatted my constant strives toward perfection and acceptance as a teenager with slews of partying. I labelled

---

1 Tagay S, Schlottbohm E, Reyes-Rodriguez ML, Repic N, Senf W. Eating disorders, trauma, PTSD, and psychosocial resources. Eat Disord. 2014;22(1):33-49. doi: 10.1080/10640266.2014.857517. PMID: 24365526; PMCID: PMC3966425.

myself as rebellious, just partying and having dumb fun like all the other kids did, like everyone said kids were supposed to. The partying didn't stop when I left home. I brushed it off, told myself this was how you were supposed to spend your time in college, but that was just another simple excuse to ignore my ED. I continuously tested my limits for consumption; I never said no to an offer to try something foreign and never carried regard for what would happen to me if the night came where I pushed myself too far. Those nights where I pushed myself almost-too far came regularly and often spun out of my control when an emotional trigger was at its core.

There are large chunks of time from my first year of college I cannot remember. My world went black and in what felt like a few moments turned into actual months going by. My room during my first year of college had a large, shared balcony that quickly became a popular hangout spot. I would guess a minimum of five people were always drinking or smoking on that porch. My substance intake was at an all-time high when I lived here. There were consecutive nights where my friends and I overindulged: we rolled several joints, ate high dosage edibles, packed a few pipes, and filled our glasses with pure liquor and no chasers. We sat in a circle on the porch and passed each item around in quick succession until every gram of weed and drop of alcohol was gone. I floated through two months of school not knowing if or how I ended up at class or back in my bed. None of this was the reaction to an obvious stressor, just a standard almost daily practice that didn't have an expiration date.

A binge born from a particular stressor was a different beast altogether. In the fall of 2013, I received news that my mother was leaving my father. After many years of failed attempts at separation, I wasn't sure if this time would stick. I learned that this time my father had threatened my mother's life (again), but also the lives of one of my brothers and sister in-law. Police arrived at my childhood home to search the premises, found the threats were real, and arrested him. I still carry this news with me today. I was heartbroken over the fact that my family history continued repeating itself, placing everyone I love in danger once again. Yet, if you were in the same room as me when I heard the news, you would think I was celebrating something joyful. I recall cheering and dancing while thanking a god I didn't believe in for finally making my family safe, which absolutely deserved a little rejoicing. But my celebratory mood didn't last long, as the complicated feelings I developed from my tenuous relationship with my father made me a fragile person. I started sinking into myself again. Anger vibrated from every pore. I felt guilty for not being more present to protect and support my family. Then, right on schedule, my emotional devolution to a sense of grief joined the party. Existing with so many simultaneous sensations grew into something too difficult to bear without any kind of comfort. I still wasn't used to reaching out to anyone as a form of consolation, and I did not yet believe that needing a friend wasn't always a burden, so I reached for something else. I filled myself with vices, running into the dark corners of drug baggies and drowning myself with bottle after bottle.

I think I sought the painful aftermath of binge drinking and substance dependency because it *was* comforting. It was almost as if the certainty of a hangover or the guaranteed agony of a drug-fueled comedown gave me joy because it was *a real example of how suffering could be temporary*. Coming out of those brief windows of misery resulted in beautiful feelings of happiness and gratitude. My body would overflow with promises to never drink again—promises I would break the next time I felt an ounce of stress or became conflicted about eating or keeping the food I ate down.

Incidentally, my alcohol and substance intake saw a drastic decrease during quarantine. For the first two weeks of quarantine, I was so overwhelmed by the state of our world, preparing to move out of a toxic living environment, moving during a pandemic (and how the hell that even works), and fearing the uncertainty of my employment status that I turned into a walking amalgamation of distress and insecurity. It was like all the anxiety and fear was enough to make me feel so numb that, in a sense, I already felt inebriated. Every day I wake up and wonder if today is the day I will lose my job and every night I lie awake hoping everyone I love is still healthy. But now some of the dust from quarantine has settled and I am starting to feel the strain from fighting my reflexive desires to engage in drinking the moment the quiet sun peeks through my blinds, signaling the start of another day I will spend searching for purpose.

Before the COVID-19 outbreak, I was in a much healthier place in terms of my ED and I felt more stable than ever before. For the past two years, I regularly binged and purged at least three days out of the week, along with undereating and committing myself to exercising after work and on the weekends, even when it meant I skipped plans with friends. This was my natural response to a painful and disturbing breakup; for years, this was my natural response to processing any kind of trauma. I find myself wondering if my recent under fueling is an unconscious reaction to processing trauma, except this time it's an external shared trauma born from a global pandemic, leaving millions of people without loved ones, job security, or a sense of hope. I spent my whole life learning how to compartmentalize and isolate as a means of survival. Self-imposed isolation became comfortable, often time even welcomed. But forced isolation is unnerving.

We are all simultaneously processing different types of traumas stemming from the COVID-19 pandemic; we are all trying to work and thrive while leaving little space to grieve. But we need to remember how to move gently. Being alive is more important than being thin. Being alive is more important than having our productivity measured through capitalism and having our worth defined through public approval. There is no need to push yourself any harder when the fluid nature of this global challenge is constantly forcing us to the brink. It feels like I'm constantly searching for answers, for a right way to survive through this, but I don't think there is any one way I can. All I know right now is this: I don't know when we'll get out of this or what it will look like when we do, but I'll be there and eager to be with all of you. I won't let isolation win anymore.

Bio: Eden Julia Sugay received their B.A. in Creative Writing from Mills College and is pursuing their MFA in Writing at University of San Francisco. Eden is Poetry Editor for Apricity Press and a reader for *Invisible City Literary Journal.* Their writing highlights their voice as a queer person of color and explores identity, relationships, and their constantly evolving natures. Their work has appeared in The Walrus, Kissing Dynamite, and Folkways Press. When Eden isn't frantically jotting half-formed thoughts on the edges of napkins, they like to fill their time dancing, baking, and exploring new ways love can manifest. Writers who quite literally give Eden life are Audre Lorde, James Baldwin, Ocean Vuong, and Ada Limón.

HEALING MY MIND

AND ACCEPTING THE ILLNESS IN MY BRAIN

by Mark Richardson

In the summer of 2019, after evaluating the options, I concluded the best way to kill myself was by jumping in front of a train. I did not want to be one of those people who attempted to end it all and failed, so approaches I deemed less likely of success (e.g., hanging, asphyxiation) were immediately discarded. Ten years earlier, my mother had died by suicide by taking pills, but I didn't have an adequate supply. A handgun seemed the most efficient approach, but I wasn't a gun person and refused to become one, even under the circumstances. And although I live in the Bay Area, I never considered jumping off the Golden Gate Bridge.

Once I zeroed in on the train, I devoured all the online articles I could find on the topic. As it turned out, quite a number of people have killed themselves by jumping in front of San Francisco's Caltrain. It's a gruesome way to go, and leaves an ugly scar on the conductors, cleaning crews, and others who witness the event and its aftermath. That dissuaded me somewhat, but not completely. I memorized the train schedules so I'd know when the express ran through Burlingame, the town where I used to live and where I planned to commit my final act. Something I've never told anyone until now is that I actually drove out to Burlingame, twice, to get the lay of the land and identify the best spot to position myself on the tracks.

I also obsessively scrolled through articles on my iPhone about Robin Williams, Anthony Bourdain, Virginia Wolff, Kate Spade, and other celebrities who had died by suicide. I wasn't romanticizing the act; it just seemed like my only logical option, and I was seeking validation.

Obviously, I didn't follow through with my plans.

As I look back, I wonder if I was truly serious or just gripped with an overwhelming suicidal ideation. What to make of it all now? Just the other week, a friend texted me: "Write about this period, brother." So here I go.

* * *

My downward turn began at my job. I worked as a marketing manager for a tech company in Silicon Valley, where I was part of a dysfunctional group. For months, team members only begrudgingly spoke to each other, causing human resources to become involved, and we all suffered through a decidedly stressful environment. Things peaked during a meeting with my manager where we screamed at each other in a tiny, windowless, steamy conference room. Afterward, I found myself experiencing acute anxiety, which manifested itself physically. I began to have trouble walking properly. My left arm hooked upward and stopped swinging as I moved, as if I was defending my side. I literally shook – my left hand and foot twitched uncontrollably. As I shuffled through the office hallways, I caught coworkers glancing at me sideways.

I also began to notice a strange smell in my nose. As these physical symptoms worsened, it created even more anxiety, until I spiraled down into such a hot mess that my wife demanded I stay home on medical leave.

I'd never before experienced anxiety or depression, but they've galloped through my family. There was my mother, but also other family members, who've struggled with suicidal thoughts. Things got so bad for my grandmother she was given electric shock therapy. I'd also had several friends who lived through debilitating bouts of depression and anxiety. Now, it seemed, it was my turn.

As my physical symptoms failed to improve, I tried to book an appointment with my doctor, but he was on a vacation, so I saw his backup instead. I explained what I was experiencing, showed him my quivering hand, and he agreed I was experiencing anxiety. He prescribed Ativan, which stopped the shaking and coated me in a blissful cocoon. When the pills ran out, I went to see my regular doctor, who had returned, seeking a fresh dose, but he wouldn't refill the prescription. He told me Ativan had awful side effects and was horribly addictive. He suggested what I really needed was to go to an outpatient facility.

For six weeks, I took an Uber to the outpatient facility – five days a week, seven hours a day. Each day was split between sessions where patients took turns talking about their problems and sessions where the counselors taught us tools to help deal with anxiety and depression. Most of the other patients had suffered experiences far worse than what I had gone through, and I watched as they benefited from the program. I didn't get better. If anything, I got worse. As we discussed our problems, my body continued to shake uncontrollably. Although it was against the rules, I was allowed to periodically go into a closed room where I'd stretch out on a sofa with a pillow between my knees and try to calm my quivering body. During formal breaks, I would go on walks, still reduced to a shuffling gait.

As the weeks slipped by, my physical condition worsened while my anxiety intensified. I began to eat less frequently and, as a result, lost a significant amount of weight. So much, my jeans no longer fit. I was certainly in no condition to return to work. As the end of the six-week period approached, I saw no improvement and became frantic.

I began to have my first suicidal thoughts.

Watching me deteriorate was terrible for my wife. Unlike me, she had no direct experience with anxiety or depression, so she began to look for another explanation. She's a nurse, and instinctually turned toward trying to find a physical cause for my symptoms. She decided I had Parkinson's disease. Obviously, I thought this was ridiculous. My friends and family and counselors all agreed. My wife persisted. She even enlisted a friend, another nurse, to support her theory.

Once, as I lay on my bed with a pillow between my knees, I yelled at them: "It's ridiculous! And what's funny is the two nurses are the ones who are misdiagnosing what is going on." They looked at each other but didn't respond.

To humor my wife, I went with her to visit my doctor. She explained her theory, and surprisingly, he didn't laugh her off but booked an appointment for me with a neurologist. My wife took me to that appointment. I was angry with her for wasting my time and was so animated I could not sit. I frantically paced in the cramped examination room as the neurologist conducted a series of tests—touching my nose, swinging my arms, moving my eyes, and snapping my fingers. As I completed the last test, I explained to the doctor what had happened to me at work and my family's history with depression, including my mother's suicide. I was so agitated that I didn't speak, but literally screamed at her, red faced.

"My wife has convinced herself of something that is obviously not true," I said. "Tell her the truth. Tell her the truth!"

The doctor leaned toward me. "You want the truth?"

"Yes!"

"You have Parkinson's disease."

At that moment, you could have knocked me over with a feather. I was so locked into my way of thinking that I didn't want to believe the diagnosis. As my wife drove us home, I turned to her and said, "That woman is a quack. When you're a hammer, you think everything is a nail. She's a neurologist, so of course she came to that conclusion." The next day, I went back to the outpatient facility and told my favorite counselor the news. She shook her head and said, "You don't have Parkinson's. You have anxiety."

There is no test that can conclusively determine whether someone has Parkinson's. After one diagnosis, it is recommended you see another doctor for a second opinion. So, I booked another appointment and my wife drove me and our kids across the bay, where a second neurologist ran me through the same tests. Her conclusion? "There is a ninety percent chance you have Parkinson's." She arranged for me to see a movement order specialist at the Stanford Neuroscience Health Center, but I would have to wait six weeks.

Sadly, the diagnosis didn't help my mental state. For starters, I still didn't believe it, at least not fully. Cognitive dissonance is a powerful thing. Despite the conclusion of two Ivy League-educated experts, I continued to tell myself my family had a history of mental illness and that's what I was experiencing. I also began to fixate on suicide.

One day, after my second trip to the Burlingame train station, I let my wife in on my morbid thoughts and told her I felt like I was dying. She was convinced all my psychological problems were connected to the Parkinson's, and said, "I'm tired of waiting for your appointment." She dropped the kids off with some friends and drove me to the emergency room at Stanford Hospital. While a doctor took my blood pressure, I prattled on about how I constantly thought about killing myself. In the emergency room, I met with a doctor who was both a neurologist and a psychologist. He had me—for a third time—do a neurological exam.

When I was finished, still stubbornly locked into my old mindset, I said, "My problem is anxiety, right?"

"You do have anxiety, but there is more going on than that. You have an illness."

"Really?"

"One hundred percent. You have Parkinson's, which explains what is happening to you."

"What do we do now?"

"We're going to put you into the Stanford Inpatient Facility."

"No," I said. "I don't want to do that. I want to go home."

"You're suicidal. I can't let you go home."

Pro tip: if you're in a hospital and don't want to be institutionalized, don't talk about suicide.

My ordeal was dreadful for my wife, who had to work, do the lion's share of the parenting, and worry about whether she'd come home and find me dead. Because of this, my sister flew in from Indianapolis and was there to greet me on the day of my discharge. She escorted me to the airport, where together we boarded a plane to Chicago, and she took me to my brother's house. I spent three weeks with my brother and his wife, eating their food, sleeping on their futon, and playing board games with their friends. It healed my mind, if not my body.

One day, while walking along the shore of Lake Michigan, my brother said to me, "There *is* something going on with you. More than just depression."

"Really?"

"Yes. I can see it."

I finally began to accept the truth and became determined to reclaim my life.

***

In September, my wife and I met with the movement disorder specialist at the Stanford Neuroscience Health Center. After yet another exam, he said in a matter-of-fact way, "Of course you have Parkinson's," confirming what my wife believed from the start. I've always known how lucky I am to be married to her, and now I feel like she saved my life. I know how frustrating it can be to know you are right about something and have nearly everyone disagree with you. Recently she told me, "I never understood why you listened to everyone else when I was the person living with you."

That day at the Neuroscience Health Center, I told the movement disorder specialist all that had happened to me—the depression, anxiety, the suicidal thoughts—and he said everything could be attributed to the disease. "If you're looking for an honorable explanation, you have it." When I told my brother that line later, he disapproved, saying, "There is nothing dishonorable about mental illness." He's right, of course. Still, hearing it from a doctor who specialized in supporting Parkinson's patients *finally* convinced my stubborn mind of the truth. What's more, I felt happy to have an answer. I imagine I'm one of the few people given a Parkinson's diagnosis who was relieved to hear the news.

* * *

Today, the sanguine feeling I had when I finally accepted my Parkinson's diagnosis has changed somewhat. Although my mental outlook has brightened, my physical condition has worsened. One of the numerous challenges I face is that the left side of my body is a mess, particularly my hand (I'm left-handed), which is stubbornly hooked like a claw and is increasingly less functional. My handwriting is atrocious, brushing my teeth is a challenge, and when I chop vegetables, I tend to mildly lose control and have tiny cut marks sprinkled on my right hand to prove it. And Parkinson's is progressive, so I can expect it to get worse. A local sports radio DJ (Ralph Barbieri), who also shared the disease, died recently, and one of his erstwhile on-air colleagues explained that the last year of his life was tough. "Parkinson's closes like a bitch," he said.

Still, I know this: I want to live! And although there is no cure for Parkinson's, my neurologist has prescribed ways to help: eat well (Mediterranean diet), get plenty of sleep, exercise, take Sinemet, and avoid stress. I worked in Silicon Valley for thirty years. That is no longer possible. For now, I'm not thinking about what lies ahead, but focusing on living each day, spending time with my wife and kids, and doing the things I enjoy, like writing.

Bio: Mark Richardson is the author of the novels *The Sun Casts No Shadow* and *Hunt for the Troll.* His short stories have appeared in numerous publications, including *Hobart*, *Fugue*, *Segue*, *Crime Factory*, and *Switchback.* Born in the Chicago area, he graduated from the University of Iowa, and promptly escaped the midwestern winters for sunny California, first living in Los Angeles and then San Francisco. Mark now lives in the East Bay with his wife, two children, and the world's cutest dog. You can find him at www.authormarkrichardson.com and @rchrdsnmark.

PERSPECTIVE, SOLITUDE, AND THE ART CONNECTION

by Emilee Prado

TO WHOM IT MAY CONCERN

I'll lead you in with an analogy: Forgoing yourself in favor of acceptance is like carving off the corners of a square peg; that round hole is accessible now, but only at the cost of stability. In this essay, I'll begin by discussing the difficulty I've had with finding a place for myself within various communities and end with how the COVID-19 pandemic—despite its atrocity—gave me permission to be comfortable with solitude.

A quick disclosure: I'm a writer, not a health or mental health professional. Any authority I claim or seem to claim regarding anxiety, depression, and/or PTSD comes only from my subjective experiences. Near the end when I discuss solitude, it is not meant to encourage any kind of repression, stark isolationism, or the rejection of outside assistance. The resources available to me have been incongruous with what I needed, so I've done a lot of bootstrap pulling. This essay's aim is to be helpful and/or useful to those who need it.

A BRIEF HISTORY OF MY ADOLESCENCE (WHO I AM AND WHERE I'M COMING FROM)

What's wrong with you?

This is a line from my childhood that has taunted me. The rhetorical question was usually spoken by my older sister. It took on different and less hostile forms when coming from others. *Weird*, *eccentric*, and *strange* (often used with endearment) have always been adjectives used in relation to my tastes and behavior. Throughout my life, I've embraced these terms, despised them, performed them, or gone to great lengths to refute them. Like most children, I thought everyone saw the world in the same way I did, so I tried to communicate things in the manner they entered my senses. Once, when trying to ask my dad about that barely perceptible flicker in all fluorescent light bulbs, I said, "Why do the lights do this?", and I rapidly blinked my eyes.

I idolized my dad, who worked as a mechanic, and this is probably why I took to building little contraptions (obstacle courses for stuffed animals, rudimentary Rube Goldberg machines, or systems of climbing ropes and swings between the two trees in my parents' backyard). These were solitary activities and were quickly dismantled before anyone could see them. I played alone so no one could call me a weirdo, but at the same time, I feared what many kids fear: that being alone makes you a loser.

I was homeschooled and brought up in an unhealthy relationship with religion (to extrapolate on this point, I would need another essay). My outsiderness was reinforced when, at age fourteen, I received the much-longed-for privilege of entering a public high school.

Although I would go on to excel academically and graduate with high honors in the top percent of my class, I was particularly terrible at one thing: making friends. A good portion of my lunch breaks were spent eating my peanut butter and honey sandwich in a bathroom stall before retreating to the library (where food wasn't allowed). Sure, I was teased or ridiculed on occasion, but I was never explicitly bullied. I hid my anxiety, smiled and was polite; others reciprocated. I wavered in and out of several groups, but any social faux pas never failed to cause a disproportionate number of tears at night.

There was a disconnect with others I couldn't understand or navigate. Part of this came from how I was raised in the world but not of it (as the church would say). I didn't understand pop-culture references and I didn't speak the right language—I was forever embarrassing myself when trying to use the local patois and slang. I should note that I also had particularly bad acne, which was in no way helpful in these early and relatively benign mental/emotional struggles.

Whether anxiety, depression, and suicidal ideation came from how I interacted with others or how I interacted with others came from my already extant brain chemistry is in the realm of the chicken and the egg. It was in university courses, though, where I learned to connect these terms with what I was feeling. I started to understand myself through the study of the sciences, and more so through the study of literature and film.

But it only got harder from there.

A (SORT OF) BRIEF INTERMISSION TO TALK ABOUT LANGUAGE

Unfortunately, the terms and concepts I learned came to me already soaked in pathology. In psychology, anxiety, depression, and PTSD are set in opposition to the normal brain. But how is it not normal to feel depressed about the inability to form deep and lasting social connections? How is it not normal to feel anxious about putting oneself into the same situation that previously begot anxiety? Or to avoid that situation altogether? How is it not normal to feel hurt and frustrated when others cannot relate to you? How is it not normal to acknowledge that death really is one way—albeit a taboo way—to escape?

We could look at what's happening here and see these ongoing responses as rational and logical given the external stimuli. Logic is frequently set up in opposition to emotion (the brain versus the heart) but anyone with a rudimentary understanding of anatomy knows the truth here – we've found a false dichotomy. Let's continue taking things apart.

Because we know that language shapes perspective, dissolving stigmas sometimes comes by way of changing the language we use. This is an ongoing progression and has evolved over the last century. Take these examples: People who die by suicide are now victims instead of criminals or sinners. Terms like *ableism* emerged to point out lack of equality in our society. Same-sex relationships are no longer called deviant behavior. The number of words we use to describe gender identity has proliferated. We've done away with the diagnosis and repurposed the (now almost laughable) 19th century term *hysteria.*

But maybe we haven't gone far enough. Talking about abstract psychological experiences and their correlating physical manifestations inside the binary of healthy vs. ill might not be the best way to move forward.

We're boxed into these terms, in part, by the desire to equate the brain with the other bodily organs and by the desire to use blameless language; it's not a person's fault if they become ill. However, ill is a negative and healthy is a positive, which leads to the assumption that ill is bad/wrong and healthy is good/right. Therefore, when I was placed in proximity to the term *mental illness,* it still felt as if someone were asking, *what's wrong with you?*

We typically construct our inner workings as horizontal goods and bads or vertical ups and downs. But what if we were able to picture them differently? (I'm open to suggestions).

Because mental and emotional experiences are deeply personal and largely incommunicable, we must settle for generalizations and labels. Experiences with depression are communicated using other abstractions (hopelessness, worthlessness, disproportionate guilt, profound grief, etc.) or by using descriptive imagery (being trapped, empty, vacuous, falling, drowning, etc.). People might have wildly different experiences with this, but we amass it under having depression. Labels are useful in some ways, but they mistakenly take what is abstract and morph it into something concrete.

The complexity of anxiety, depression, and PTSD, etc., their potent physical symptoms, and their tendency to dominate the emotional landscape is what differentiates them from more transient negative emotions such as jealousy, sorrow, longing, or fear. However, by giving a specific form to anxiety or depression or PTSD, each of these experiences can then be called *it* (a word that stands for the representation of an inanimate object). We're taking what we feel and giving it more tangibility and permanence as a thing we have. For example, someone might say: I've felt hopeless and empty since my spouse died. Rather than: I've had hopelessness and emptiness since my spouse died. Likewise, someone might say: I had PTSD after I was raped. Rather than: I felt PTSD after I was raped.

In making things too concrete, we take what is ethereal and add burdensome weight. On the other hand, sometimes personal accounts praise the label/ diagnosis for pinning down something that was otherwise too vague. For some, the label shaped the concrete thing into an opponent, a thing that could be battled. The label thus enables the metaphorical dragon. Familiar weapons for those in the know are usually a combination of personal strategies, pharmaceuticals, CBT or other therapy, dietary changes, and/or self-analysis. There have been reports of victories.

Maybe the dragon slaying method is empowering and really works for some people, but it didn't work for me. I felt I'd been dropped with the weight of having something (something wrong with me) then presented with the image of a monstrous beast I was supposed to defeat. This confrontation left me feeling as if I were one in the multitude of brave knights who was about to be immolated or eaten before the real hero appears.

I don't like to give my negative psycho-physiological experiences so much clout as to say I'm at battle with them; I prefer pacifism to being a soldier in an endless war. Maybe instead I could say: I've experienced occasional and concentrated amounts of intense psycho-physiological distress? Anyway, it was access to art and solitude that helped me generate self-compassion and shift the language I used to create my perceptions. More on that later.

MY CONTINUING SOCIAL/EMOTIONAL DIFFICULTIES

We'll pick up between 2009 and 2013. I was in my early twenties, at university. I was working on a triple major: Film Studies, Literature, and the neuroscience track of Psychology. How I'd turn these into a career wasn't at the forefront of my mind. I was too busy unearthing vital information about how totally cool and bizarre it was to be a human.

In psych classes, I learned the term *Introvert*. I learned the term *Highly Sensitive Person*. I learned what was covered under the term *sexual assault.* I learned to call the disruptive physical/emotional states I oscillated between anxiety and depression. I realized that it could be called abnormal to have occasional bouts of what seemed to be suffocation, and that it could be called abnormal to go through phases of not being able to feel any feeling at all. I also learned about neurotransmitters and how certain chemicals influenced the brain.

I tried to take control of what I'd now come to see as faulty wiring and I followed the only template I knew, the one with the battle imagery. I was put on Citalopram and Alprazolam after a brief consultation with a general practitioner. I used these pills and my weapons of knowledge and swung and wrenched and fought. When this did not work, I tried repression and denial. I sometimes reverted to the well-hidden self-harm I'd started at age eleven or twelve.

By university, I'd become slightly better at socializing. I stuck with the group of friends/roommates randomly assigned to me via freshman year dorm room proximity and dutifully tagged along to parties and bars. I had some great times, but often I just participated. I would feign/perform enjoyment of drinking games, loud music, and/or dancing. Inside classrooms and lecture halls, I'd occasionally find enthusiasts for academics like myself, but I was too soggy with inferiority to try to befriend them. There was still a social disconnect; I still thought I was a resident of loserdom.

I continued to be embarrassed by the response some of my stories provoked and this perpetuated some of my solipsistic self-loathing. Here's an example. I don't remember exactly what was going on, but it was a casual gathering, there was probably booze and weed. This is what I shared:

In the fall semester of my freshman year of high school, I needed to get a sports physical in order to join the cross-country team. My mom took me to an affordable clinic, and it happened to be in a mobile trailer in a church parking lot (I didn't think this part was weird, but my listeners did). I went in by myself, got the form signed, done. I had no idea that it wasn't standard practice for a doctor to remove his gloves or ask a teenage girl getting a sports physical to pull down her pants and underwear. At dinner that night, I mentioned to my family how I thought it was unnecessary for the doctor to examine my vagina. I was reprimanded. My parents told me, "Don't talk like that at the dinner table."

I shared this story in response to comments made about a sexual assault that had been on the news. I argued that it wasn't right to call my experience sexual assault because I'd felt mildly annoyed, not assaulted. To my surprise, my friends were sort of repelled. Someone said something like, "How did you not know he was molesting you?" And—no joke—someone said: "What's wrong with you?" I became ashamed, not about what happened, but for not knowing—at fourteen—that what had happened was wrong.

The doctor in the trailer would not be my only non-consensual sexual encounter. The assault that occurred later in my twenties was physically violent. By then, I had no hesitations or doubts about the wrongness of the act.

Although I was struggling emotionally and socially, I stopped taking the Citalopram and Alprazolam because the pills made me constantly drowsy and—with nothing else at hand—I needed to be able to thrive on academics. Courses in philosophy, astronomy, and earth science forced me to reckon with the falseness of the religion I'd been sloughing off over the years. In theory courses, I learned about deconstruction, semiotics, the postmodern, surrealism, and the sublime, all which impacted my worldview. I learned about absurdism. I wondered about Albert Camus' one serious philosophical problem: Deciding whether or not life is worth living.

Like the absurdists, I thought it was reasonable and logical to acknowledge life as pointless, but this didn't make me hopeless; it fascinated me. I longed for discourse outside classrooms, but my conversation topics were usually incompatible with the vibe of the party scene.

Unfortunately, burgeoning knowledge partnered with my continued social dissonance and an uptick in negative experiences led to continued furtive self-harm and more than one secret plan for suicide. It was around then that I also fell in love for the first time. However, the incongruity between social performances and genuine intimacy turned out to be precarious territory.

I felt myself turned over to my university's counseling and psychological services, a place that would pathologize me. I'd tried to talk with a therapist on two separate occasions, but both made me feel judged which prevented me from returning. (Also note that therapy requires a healthy social connection between two people, the exact thing I was terrible at forming). My aversion to traditional help was further complicated by my knowledge of the 72-hour-hold—I'd have to lie about feeling suicidal, so what was the point of going in? I'd seen the results of the so-called help people had received because suicide and substance abuse run in my family (one of my relatives had died by suicide in the dorms of the very university I was attending). I was further wary because I knew of others who had gone through treatments like "pray-the-gay-away."

I had a stigma against the mental health care system because I didn't see it as the authority figure it claimed to be. In part, I was convinced that it was a money-and-power-hungry institution, which overwrote any humanitarian aspect. Furthermore, I saw the root of my problems as existential, not clinical. In part, I was trapped in a psychological storm because there were questions I needed answered: What is human consciousness? What's the overall purpose of life on planet earth? Why do some babies die of cancer? Why exactly should I wait to die until sometime after I've gone grey and retired from my nine-to-five?

I was probably right in thinking that the person on the other end of the line couldn't answer these questions, so I ignored the follow-up calls from psychiatric services.

TO QUIT OR TO PLAY A DIFFERENT WAY

I suspect unanswerable questions and the limit of human knowledge will remain difficult for some of us to contend with, but I've settled for ways to avoid drowning in them. And today, at thirty, if someone were to ask *what's wrong with you?* I could reply honestly: *nothing*.

I've continued to avoid professional help (this is not an explicit recommendation, please recall the disclaimer in the intro). However, I did not come to a more peaceful existence unassisted. The main people I have to thank are ones I've never spoken to – academics, writers, researchers, filmmakers, and scientists—not to ignore or forget to thank the people in my life (especially teachers) who gave me or led me to certain sources and/or ideas.

I've recently read about the statistically significant positive effects of art therapy and—although I can't attest to what methods are used by professionals—I'm comfortable advocating for it here because of my experiences with art itself. It's artists who seem most adept at dealing with the unknowable. I've come to see works of art as intermediaries – art exists in the abstract and people summon it into this world via their craft (for me it's writing, sometimes visual art, and/or guitar). This means that art occupies the same ethereal space where feelings reside. With works of art, mental/emotional experiences can be made concrete not via a pathology (recall: to *have* anxiety/depression/PTSD) but via an artistic medium. There may be an extant term for this type of manifestation, but I call it the art connection. If this seems too abstract, it probably is. But perhaps embracing the abstract would lessen some of society's mental strife.

The art connection also helped me to discover a minimalist lifestyle. I was able to help maintain psychic equilibrium by keeping a balance between consumption, creation, and rest. Consumption, here, meaning any intake: media or text, natural resources, generosity received, etc. And creation, here, meaning any sort of personal output including attitude, art, work, volunteering, etc. The balance takes on diverse forms as long as I feel as if I'm giving back the same amount I take.

Co-emerging with the art connection for me was a growing body awareness that came from better regulating my diet, how I exercised, and by learning meditation. Each of these things have been notably praised in mental health literature. I won't take the time to go into further detail here other than to say this: If you've struggled psychologically, remember that the brain is an organ. It might behoove you to know what's in your food and how your body responds to it, and again, to balance the input and output of energy.

What solidified further change in me was 2020, the year I received societal permission to be alone. Isolation and social distancing transmuted my psychological landscape and abated many of my struggles. I was privileged enough to be single and living alone when the world went into lockdown. Suddenly, I saw the things that disturbed me become normalized. It was fine to be anxious about the state of our global society. Depression was acceptable, too. All of us were traumatized. It was normal to be homeschooled (for a year or two at least). Moreover, there was nothing wrong with being alone—in fact, I was helping others by isolating myself from them. Despite the aching compassion I felt for the horrors people were facing, I settled into a new contentment with myself. The pandemic erased what had caused so much contention for me. I used to think it was necessary to be social, so I fought to do so and frequently failed, not only at socializing, but also at honoring my independence. By the time others went back out to congregate, I no longer felt that social isolation was forced on me; it was a newfound choice of lifestyle.

I am, of course, neither the first to tout the powers of solitude nor to use an essay to demonstrate the stigma against it. You probably already know that being alone does not equal loneliness. Loneliness comes with negative impacts, but solitude is restorative. Loneliness usually has something to do with feeling misunderstood, but hopefully these last few paragraphs have scratched the surface of how changing the relationship with the self can mitigate perceived ostracization. Furthermore, by acknowledging the abstractness of human feelings and accepting that language cannot thoroughly communicate our inner world we admit that emotions, psychological reactions/processes, and social well-being are in constant flux. Recognizing this intangibility can invite release.

Bio: Emilee Prado is currently embracing solitude in Tucson, Arizona. Her publications include a variety of nonfiction as well as experimental, narrative, and hybrid fiction. Her work is forthcoming in several anthologies and appears in *Cincinnati Review*, *Hobart*, *CRAFT*, *Subnivean,* and elsewhere. Find out more at emileepradoauthor.com.

ESCAPE

Elizabeth White

I grew up in a small town of backyards, cul-de-sacs, and quiet, winding roads. Nestled in the Hudson Valley of upstate New York (the upstate distinction being dependent on whether you were from the city or not), our house opened to an empty field and the silhouette of a sloping green mountain. As a child, I liked to imagine it was the sleeping form of a mighty dragon that would one day take me away. There was no destination in mind, no navigation chart in hand. Only away.

All my life, I dreamed of escaping it. At first, according to my earliest memories, few and foggy as they are, escape was synonymous with adventure. A young explorer in the making, I yearned to discover the potential and possibilities the big vast world had to offer.

I settled for the forests and farmlands in the Empire State. The place of my birth was defined by green hills and valleys, divided by wide rivers and winding gravel roads, enclosed by green-topped mountains, low and wide and many. My three brothers and I grew up in a time when children were allowed, nay encouraged, to go outside and play. So long as you were back by the dinner bell, the day was yours. Behind our messy backyard, always littered with abandoned toys or my parent's random tools or gardening equipment (and later, a collection of broken hot tubs that were the result of my father's atrocious haggling skills) there was a stretch of woods. In those residential areas, we were forced to listen to the adults, but in that crop of trees, we could be free.

The woods looked like a solid wall, a clear border marking the boundary between the cut grass of our backyard and the untamed brush beyond. Filled with deciduous trees, pricker bushes, and animal paths, it was less than a mile long, and couldn't have been more than a quarter mile deep. Yet to a child, the small, wooded area was a great unknown that stretched without end. And within it, laid treasures untold.

It was home to a swamp we skirted around, fearing it might be toxic, secret groves we fashioned into forts, animal paths that twisted and turned. The groundhog hole on the small hill led to the center of the clearing on the other side. The landing near the swamp we covered in those rubber puzzle-piece mats until someone stole them. There were bushes with red berries my brother always said were poisonous and the occasional sighting of high school stoners looking for a secluded place to get high.

It was wild, but not dangerous. More comforting than the walls of my small room. One afternoon it was a battlefield littered with nerf bullets. The next, the home to multiple forts, one for each of us. The abandoned building site of a failed treehouse. The uncharted territory where we adventurers would stake our claim.

That was the fleeting part of my life defined by innocence. Life was not carefree; I was just naive to what sort of cares existed. The way children ought to be. During those few blissful years, life simply unfolded and opened. It was full of potential and possibilities, and my dream world began and ended in those woods.

As years passed, the town grew and the woods shrank. The field on the other side of Main Street was replaced with tract housing in the shape of a horseshoe. On both sides of our house, new neighbors cut into the woods to extend their backyards. Next door, in the now cleared extension of their manicured lawn, they constructed a wooden playset they rarely ever used. Two houses down, they cleared the untamed bush, destroying a path that skirted the southern edge of the woods to erect a graveyard for old, abandoned cars.

They cut down my safe space to extend their own. The natural world sacrificed for more cul-de-sacs and cookie-cutter houses. The woods became collateral damage to the American Dream.

And while I didn't know it at the time, the childlike innocence I found there would be torn down, too. By different means, perhaps, but taken from me all the same.

It would be a very long time until any semblance of it would be reclaimed.

* * *

Existence had been unkind to me early on, and it wasn't long until I found myself unsuited for it. Faced with a crash course in the evils of the world that I could neither process nor understand, my little young brain decided it was easiest to disassociate. I spent my teenage years yearning for a different life, or to be a different person, though my biggest wish was to find a wormhole in my closet that led me to a faraway land with magic of some sort or another. I did not care for my reality, so I resorted to escaping it.

Deep depression made me insular, almost agoraphobic. I preferred fictional worlds accessed in my own home, books read and movies watched from my bedroom. People would invite me to venture out and I would decline, rinse, and repeat until, eventually, they would stop inviting me anywhere at all. Then I used the fact that I wasn't getting invited as proof as to why I shouldn't go anywhere. Thoughts of being around other people sent spikes of anxiety through my system, so jarring that all I wanted to do was be elsewhere yet found myself incapable of leaving. The boundaries of my life continued to shrink, smaller and smaller until they consisted of my house, school, dance studio, and the car that took me from one to the other.

But who needed the real world with all its dark and dreary scenery and monsters hiding in plain sight, when there were so many other worlds to stretch your legs in? Most of these worlds also featured dark and dreary scenery, and monsters hiding in plain sight. But at least in fictional ones, the bad guys were revealed and defeated in the end.

In online video games like *Everquest* and *World of Warcraft*, I didn't just explore a new world, I became a different person. I changed my face, my shape, my race. I could be someone pretty, and small, and strong—everything I believed I wasn't. And most of the time, I wasn't focused on raiding and leveling like my brothers. As a wood elf, I would pretend one of the empty houses in the city in the trees was my own. In a larger city, I set up shop in an abandoned building, selling drinks and pretending I was a pub owner.

I fell deeper and deeper into escapism, yet the sad irony was that I had kept myself stuck at the site of my trauma. I could hear it with every creak of the floorboards, feel it in the damp chill of the basement, sense it in the dark of night. Reminders of my sexual abuse were always there, swirling in the dust, seeping from the pipes, riding the damp chill of the basement's stone walls.

And even when given an opportunity, I did not leave. Part of me didn't want to or didn't see the point. If your own home isn't safe, what is? When the person that's supposed to love and protect you most lets you down, who can you trust? Besides, the rot of what happened was already within me, inseparable from me. So, it didn't matter where I went in the world, the desolation would only follow.

But not to these other worlds. The scope of personal suffering was dwarfed by the rise and fall of kingdoms or the quest to overthrow an evil tyrant in a world filled with wizards, magic swords, and fancy ladies who could compel anyone to tell the truth. What were my problems compared to the pain of my best friend becoming my greatest enemy, both of us pursuing peace in gravely different ways? Trying to figure out the past of an orphan boy who transforms into a dragon and robs from the rich with blue-haired and half-feline friends allowed me to outrun my own issues, if only for a while.

Besides, obsessing over the trials and tribulations of fictional characters made it easier to forget my own. When I was immersed in other people's stories, I could forget the ones I was telling myself of my worthlessness, my shame, my secrets.

Most of that obsession took place in the *Suikoden* universe. A Japanese role-playing series of empires and city-states, island nations, of personal betrayal and national triumph. I rallied countries and clans together to battle evil or misguided powers with the help of 108 friends and magical runes that unleashed immense power on the world. I explored an unknown world and histories and cultures unlike my own. I created my own home and filled it with friends and allies. My journey from naive youth to a powerful leader unfolded to a magnificent and sweeping soundtrack.

Escapism felt like the only healthy outlet for my emotions, which were chaotic and confusing, and mostly painful. When a character sacrificed themselves, saving me from a painful death, I cried. When a best friend escaped capture and found his way back to the group, I was elated. When I defeated the evil empire and achieved the perfect ending, resurrecting my fallen mentor, I was triumphant. These felt like normal reactions. They made sense, and I felt in control of them in a way that I didn't in my personal life, where my body exhibited strange and uncontrollable reactions to triggers I didn't know were there, or why.

It also wasn't something I shared with other people. Growing up, being a nerd wasn't cool, especially as a girl. I didn't fit in to begin with, so I didn't want to give anyone else ammunition to isolate me further. I was always weird and antisocial and awkward. Did I really want to be considered a dork or a nerd, too? I kept it a secret, just like everything else I was ashamed of.

By focusing my energy on being someplace else, and being someone else, I lost out on my formative years. I could not form relationships, whether platonic or romantic. I never learned to open up to people, preferring to keep my emotions locked away where they couldn't consume me or anyone within lash-out radius. I emerged from puberty, awkward in my own skin, both naive and knowing. The former to the joy life could bring, the latter to the pain of it.

Not that it was all bad. Video games really beef up your vocabulary. For instance, I knew the word corpse before any of my elementary school classmates. Fantasy literature and the names of the spells in *Everquest* really helped me understand Shakespeare's twang. My English teacher once called me a "Shakespearean goddess," which I still count as one of the greatest compliments I've ever received.

Of course, ignoring the source of your shame doesn't make it go away. It just sits and stews, like gum at the bottom of your shoe. It lurks, waits, and accumulates, ready to emerge when you least expect or desire it.

***

At the age of 18, I left home for the first time, journeying northwest across New York along Route 81, past roadway diners and small sleepy towns with names that were either simultaneously uninspired and descriptive or borrowed from some minor English lord: Peaksville, Elkland, Windsor, etc.

When I landed in Buffalo, a chilly and somewhat forgotten city on the country's northern edge, I hoped the more miles I put between myself and the birthplace of my problems, the lighter the burden of them would be. The Queen City had the flatness and odd vernacular of a midwestern town that somehow got plucked from the breadbasket. Students from all over the state, as well as a few international and out-of-state kids, emerged on campus in the dog days of summer to embark on the next steppingstone of the American Dream: college.

I had no interest in this dream as described to me. A large part of me had no grand hopes or ambitions for my future because I didn't really believe I had one. The life ahead of me was a nebulous thing, murky and obscured by an overwhelming sense of futility. Sure, I had a major picked out, English, but I did not see myself as the next voice of a generation. I saw nothing for me in the future that I didn't already have in the present. Anger, bitterness, resentment, despair. Mostly, I went to college because it was expected of me and because it gave me an excuse to get away.

But there was another part of me, the stubbornly optimistic one that kept trying to spot some light at the end of the inky tunnel. The part that kept hoping for more. It wondered if this could be my chance at a fresh slate, to put unpleasantness behind me and be someone new. And not just by tweaking my appearance to align with societal beauty standards and giving myself bitching magical powers as I had done in video games. Real change. Add a dash of openness and optimism, reduce bitchy and sullen behavior, take out the messy gunk of childhood trauma, and voilá, the new and improved me.

This was easier said than done. Growth doesn't come from paving over your problems, and the process of healing takes bravery I hadn't tapped into yet. The setting might have changed, but the things I carried remained, weighing me down, poking out from my periphery like the culprit hiding in plain sight of the whodunit.

When I first settled into my dorm, filled with excitement and nerves to begin this grand formative experience *Superbad* and *Animal House* had prepared me for, I remember telling my roommate that I didn't drink or party much. This was true – until it wasn't.

Since I had few friends or romantic connections in high school, I had little practice in the social situations that came with being a college student. In the early days, drinking became a social crutch, something to loosen inhibitions and quiet the inner critic that was providing mean-girl commentary on my every move. With each drink I had, the weight of things lifted, my tongue loosened, my smile sneaked through the suspicious bars that often held it down.

It wasn't until my sophomore year that drinking became something like a need. My father died at the end of my freshman year, and I had hoped the pain he caused would die with him. Instead, it only became worse. I did not magically become happy and shame-free, or learn to manage my emotions, or stop lying by omission. Everything was the same, except now there was a gnawing hole where the root of it all used to be.

My plan was to fill that emptiness with FourLoko, 99 Apples, and whatever shudder-inducing ingredients comprised frat party jungle juice. This method yielded results. At first. When I was drunk, I felt okay being myself, I didn't automatically see deceit and cruelty and suspicion behind every face in the crowd, and most importantly, I could forget.

Alcohol allowed me to be someone else. The party girl who was unapologetic, wild, as deep as a Red Solo cup, someone in on the joke that was herself. Because if you're laughing, too, people can only laugh with, not at, you. My friends even gave this drunk alter ego a name: Fritz. I desperately wanted to be that person. To be the person who could go to a party and just talk to strangers, not automatically assume everyone hated her, and mentally list the reasons why. To have a healthy sex life, one unmoored by trauma. Most of all, I wanted to be normal.

Despite my best efforts, the hole never filled. Every morning I woke up with an emptiness in my gut, desperate and aching to be doused once more. No matter how many one-night-stands, fights I picked to unleash misplaced aggression, and no matter how satiated I felt from one act of instant gratification to the next, it hungered for more. And I was more than willing to feed it.

I spent four years being the drunk girl, wading in the shallow end because that's as far as I would allow my emotional or romantic connections to go. A kid from my high school once told me that he was always happy to see me at a party because that meant he would never be the drunkest person in the room. I smiled a genuine smile in response and told him I was more than happy to assist him in that regard. Because I was.

Throughout the next four years, I had the capacity to be the improved version of myself. But I didn't want to put in the work. I wanted the world, the people around me, the situations I found myself in, to do it for me. I wanted all the benefits without any of the bother.

When it came to choosing between someone who cared for me or a string of meaningless one-night stands, I chose the latter. If my options were owning up to my mistakes or lying to get myself out of a sticky situation, I opted for my old, toxic defense mechanisms.

Fritz helped – until she didn't. She was both an escape and a punishment. I treated other people, and myself, poorly, and woke up with more reasons to be ashamed, angry, and lonely. When you never stop piling reasons to hate yourself on top of each other, it's harder to see what lies at the bottom.

***

When college ended, I drove home, past the same diners and towns, changed, but not in the way I hoped. The future looked no clearer or brighter than when I left all those years ago. Worse perhaps, as I returned to the same home I was desperate to leave. My father was gone, but his specter remained, and the ghosts of my plethora of misdeeds were soon to join him.

For the next few years, I would still drink in excess, make self-destructive choices, and push away anyone who dared to get close to me. But eventually, I reached a point of diminishing returns. The fleeting happiness of my escapism was nothing compared to the suffering I felt by just existing. I felt broken. I was the abandoned car in the graveyard, the villain you want to destroy at the end of the game, the pathetic drunk you laugh at with your friends.

Internalized pain is one hell of a master of disguise. No matter what I did to make it go away, to forget it or pretend it didn't happen or didn't matter, the trauma only adapted and evolved. Trying to escape only prolonged the inevitable.

So, one day, sitting on the deck in my backyard, staring into the woods which seemed so small and feeble now, I made a choice. I called a therapist, and when she asked me why I called, I told her the truth. I had two choices left: face the trauma I had been avoiding my whole life, or end up dead, one way or another.

And it was only then that my true escape began.

Bio: Elizbeth White (she/her/hers) is a millennial copywriter who lives in Washington, DC. She has been published online at *Oddball Magazine* and was a featured fiction reader at Inner Loop and Writers and Words, literary communities in Washington, DC, and Baltimore, MD, respectively. Her interests include the tangled web of the human heart and the folly that often defines its actions.

THE BODY AS RECLUSE:

A LYRIC ESSAY

by Alton Melvàr M Dapanas

> *"The line between insanity and mysticism is thin; the line between reality and unreality is thin. Liminality as a spiritual concept is all about the porousness of boundaries."*
>
> —*from 'Beyond the Hedge,'*
> The Collected Schizophrenias: Essays,
> *Esmé Weijun Wang*

i. Aimlessly switch from Amazon Prime to Netflix to HBO Go as you shift your weight on the couch. *Something to distract me,* you say to yourself, too loudly. So loud that you feel embarrassed, like a kid caught with a broken vase. But you're alone, you've always been. Grab the remaining half-bottle of Heineken from the case. Ants are now feasting over crumbs of pizza and smear of catsup. This disarray, this tiny chaos is what you hate. Restore a semblance of order, type in "FoodPanda, grocery, 6pm" in your Google Keep Notes.

ii. Funes from Jorge Luis Borges's story "Funes, His Memory," began his explanation with "I, myself, alone…" or consider Henrik Ibsen's *En Folkefiende* where Thomas Stockmann proclaimed his epiphany, "It is this, let me tell you—that the strongest man in the world is he who stands most alone."

Indian philosopher and monk Shantideva, too, talked of self-mastery in *The Way of the Bodhisattva*:

> Relinquishing all other aspirations,
> Focusing myself on one intent alone,
> I'll strive to still my mind,
> And, calming it, to bring it to subjection.

Several "friends" from your deleted Facebook account, as far as you remember, titled their photo album of selfies, "me, myself, and I." Maybe these people mastered their "selves" – the ones with healthy selfhood.

iii. In a 2020 study published in the *Journal of Affective Disorders*, Filipino psychologists found out that 25% of Filipinos had "moderate-to-severe anxiety, one-seventh reported moderate-to-severe stress levels and one-sixth reported moderate-to-severe depression." WHO Philippines, in an infographic, advises people like you "to talk to a mental health professional or someone you trust." More recent research in the *Asia Pacific Journal of Public Health*, *Traumatology*, and *International Psychogeriatrics*, more or less, maintained the same trend.

Another 2020 study in the *Social Psychiatry and Psychiatric Epidemiology* estimated 6 million Filipinos suffer from depression and/or anxiety, making mental illness the "third most common disability" in the country and hailing the Philippines as "the country with the third highest rate of mental health problems in the Western Pacific region." Despite this, according to a recent study in the *British Journal of Psychiatry International*, "only 3–5% of the total health budget is spent on mental health."

As of August 2020, Manila-based National Center for Mental Health noted an alarming spike of suicide-related calls in their hotline.

iv. *Didn't they say it comes as a black dog-shaped smoke? To you, it comes as a hovering voice, a litany of sins.*

v. Growing up in a culture that celebrates collectivism, where pakikisama, social harmony, is the cultural ideal, a part of you is thankful. You despised the noise, the crowds. A journalist from a TV network that the fascist government has shut down insists on using "physical distancing" over "social distancing." You do not agree with her. You've been distant to people even as a kid.

"Do you want to live as a monje?" your outgoing half-Spaniard grandfather would ask. In an undergraduate Nature Writing elective, you studied *Walden*, where Thoreau wrote, "it [is] wholesome to be alone."

But the bourgeois in you hates that the nearest 7-Eleven now closes at 9 pm. Some of your favorite restaurants have closed for months, too; a few for good. You mostly dine alone. *You want to disappear.*

vi. In *Tsurezuregusa*, or *Essays in Idleness*, late 13th century Japanese Buddhist monk Yoshida Kenkō pondered, "There is nothing finer than to be alone with nothing to distract you." You love the ruminative quality of thought embedded in classical East Asian writings—haibun (poem-in-prose), zuihitsu (essay), kikobun (travelogue), and nikki (diary).

Predating the Western diarists by eight centuries, Ennin, Sei Shōnagon, Abutsu-ni, Sarashina, Matsuo Basho, and Lady Izumi wrote several nikki. Their sense of inwardness and interiority, to you, is beau idéal, unlike your countrymen, extroverted, too-hospitable nationalists.

You wish someone will quote Kenkō in the submissions to journals you edit and read for. *Our previous issue thematically discussed this*, you remind the others in the masthead via Slack. Deep down, you're a closeted escapist, you detest being reminded of what's actually happening, Pisces-style derangement.

vii. In *The Situation and the Story: The Art of the Personal Narrative*, Vivian Gornick problematized the I-persona's aloneness in highbrow literary prose. In fiction, it's "truth-speaking," citing Dostoyevsky and Beckett, but in nonfiction, such is taken as an "artifice [that] is unacceptable" and "foolishly self-dramatizing." Gornick then mentioned European memoirists who have perfected solving "this intractable writing problem": Beryl Markham, Marguerite Duras, W.G. Sebald.

In Jean-Jacques Rousseau's *Les rêveries du promeneur solitaire,* parallelism was drawn between societal banishment and the choice of self-exile, to choose everyday solitude. In a sea of writings that only discuss one or the other and never both, this was a refreshing take from centuries ago.

viii. Sister Jude, the character portrayed by the unparalleled Jessica Lange in the Gothic camp anthology series *American Horror Story: Asylum,* declares, "Mental illness is the fashionable explanation for sin."

Despite massive campaigns by advocates from the private sectors and nongovernment organizations, Filipino society remains, in terms of mental health—and everything else—conservative. Occasionally, you will hear news of mentally ill people being imprisoned, secluded, even tied to a rope or chains inside a room or outdoors, by their own families. The current right-wing dictator himself, along with his fascist regime, adds to the stigma and subscribes to an outdated rhetoric to the point of calling his political rivals "buang," crazy.

Your therapist said that the results of the Davidson Trauma Scale say you're heading towards post-traumatic fatigue, exhaustion, not recovery.

ix. *Didn't they say it comes as a black dog-shaped smoke? To you, it comes as a hovering voice, a litany of sins.*

x. A fragment of a memory:

For the earth hour in 2019, you stood on the edge of Ysalina bridge, all of the city a pitch-black acreage of noise. Earlier, a threat of impending rain, a changing tint of bruised light suffused the sky. Your eyes drift to the horizon. Muted thunder rumbled. *Foreshadowing and Proppian prolepsis right there,* you thought. In your mind's eye, a hypothetical headline, something about paying for sins committed, something about a literal poetic justice.

Back in college, you used to have a crush on a guy from the Finance program. The crush went on for a few years, whether you're in a relationship or not. In your last year as a student council volunteer during the enrollment week, you saw him pass by, in deep thought. *Had a bad day for sure. Fight with a girlfriend?* That was the last time you'd see him. A day after, the whole university will be shocked to learn the news that he jumped off from the third story of a mall. A radio commentator would proclaim, despite having zero credentials to do so, that he was mentally ill. At the local pre-primetime newscast, a cousin of his would be interviewed, his exact words: "Tell my mother I love her." In the newspaper, he is reduced to a term, a "mall jumper."

xi. Inside the fridge are almost empty jars of pickled spices and relishes, cartons of almond milk, a bunch of fruits and vegetables you forgot to eat or cook, blocks of tofu. *I used to be the home-maker type,* you thought. Some are turning almost brown, but you have plans: banana for banana bread, vine spinach for a smoothie, grapes with soy yogurt for popsicles, sweet potato for fries.

This is not because you're a miser. This is because you have a hard time letting go, rotten fruit or not.

xii. Canadian poet-academic Alison Calder defines "deep mapping" as a special form of "vertical travel [and place-based] writing" which involves "autobiography… archeology, folklore, reportage, climate" and questions the binaries of the historical/contemporary, the political/poetic, the factual/fictional, the discursive/sensual. Unlike picturesque and romantic travel/place writing, this scientific travel/place writing emphasizes *verticality*, starts with the surface and ultimately uncovers what's beneath it.

And yet, cultural geography questions the notion that maps are "scientifically neutral." Jeanne Garane, in *Géographies discursives: l'écriture de l'espace et du lieu en français,* argues that the act of mapping places are shaped by the dominant forces in cultural production as cartographers are prone to placing their own territory as the center of their map, a classic example of ethnocentricity.

And yet, Maggie Nelson, in *Bluets*, wrote, "One can wander about the landscape looking for clues, amassing evidence, but even the highest pile never seems to decide the case."

xiii. Catastrophizing, mind-reading, and emotional reasoning, according to Cognitive Behavioral Therapy, are three of the many forms of distorted thinking. At least once a week, you'd wake up at 3 in the morning to check your email and inbox of other socials, as if anticipating The Bad News—you don't know what exactly it is but you know it is coming your way. On countless nights, you even dreamt of receiving the news.

This morning, you decide to count the hangers and arrange them by the colors of the rainbow, which was frustrating because all you have are black and gray ones. Last week, it was the empty mason jars and Tupperwares. A rope catches your attention.

xiv. It was only in 1973 when the American Psychiatric Association removed "homosexuality" from the DSM list of mental illness.

It was only in 2017 when the Danish parliament legislated to remove transgenderism as a form of mental illness.

You neither identify as "homosexual" nor Danish.

xv. *Didn't they say it comes as a black dog-shaped smoke? To you, it comes as a hovering voice, a litany of sins.*

xvi. Wearing face masks meant anonymity, blending in, being able to disappear in a crowd. But it is the island life you missed—particularly being unknown even without a mask. In one of your prose poems published in a literary journal in Berlin, you'd write:

You think about the escape from previous lives, an essential task to save the self from the city that swarmed on your banishment. Outside your apartment back in college, a man sells colorful balloons to a boy who keeps on clutching his mother's bosom, a sleepless student nurse in white is on the way to hospital duty, and there, at the cul-de-sac sidewalk, an alley of stalls of street food like caked pig's blood and unhatched duck embryo. Outside your favorite secondhand bookstore, the pharmacy you frequent, a parking lot where you jog, a notorious inn. This was your city and its attendant histories.

But here in this sun-rinsed island town, in your room, by the window, staring at the empty bird cage hanging by a topiary, an absence of breeze, just still air, still life.

xvii. You came across Low Theory as proposed by queer scholar J Halberstam, who urged the LGBTQIA+ community and its allies to rethink the preference of committing "to restoring the gay subject to history and redeeming the gay self" (products of, in the words of Halberstam, "liberal histories [that] build triumphant political narratives with progressive stories of improvement and success") over "embracing the incoherent, the lonely, the defeated, and the melancholic formulations of selfhood" (which, to Halberstam, is the role of "radical histories on legacies of failure and loneliness as the consequences of homophobia and racism and xenophobia").

"Do not appear if you do not want to disappear," goes one of Foucault's most quoted lines. *You want to disappear.*

xviii. The Middle English word recluse comes from the Old French reclure ('enclose') which in turn, is rooted from the Latin word claudere ('to shut').

But sometimes, you cannot turn to language. In your native tongue, there is no word for "introvert." "Words / I speak return lonely," wrote Filipino queer modernist poet José Garcia Villa.

xix. Instead of more concrete measures like faster vaccine rollout and more aggressive contact-tracing, the national government mandated wearing of face shields on top of face masks. CNN Philippines headlines give you migraines. The national economy is at its worst since 1947. "The world's longest and strictest lockdown," wrote *The Telegraph*.

You stopped listening to the daily briefings over local TV from the mayor of your home city. You applaud his policies, but you don't need his reminders.

xx. In *The Best American Travel Writing 2017*, lesbian poet Elizabeth Lindsey Rogers confronts in her essay the tensions between her American individual autonomy versus guanxi, the expectation of societal cohesiveness in Shanxi province in northeastern China where she had a teaching stint. She reminisces,

"Why is she not coming out here?" I heard someone ask Ben on the other side of my door. "Is she sad about something?

Why is she alone?" The word alone in Mandarin can be translated in various ways. The expression I heard on the other side of my door, traveling by myself on a train, or walking down the street solo was *yi ge ren*. *Yi* is "one"; *ge* is a kind of counting word, placed between a number and an object. And *ren* means "person" or "people." The expression "Are you *yi ge ren*?" when translated literally is "Are you one person?" In context, though, I began to understand this as a way of asking, "Are you on your own? Are you alone?"

xxi. In an e-numan (electronic + inuman, drinking session) with high school friends, everyone looked different. The extroverted ones, you've observed, tend to be openly distressed, giving off loud SOS vibe. The introverts like you were built for prolonged isolation.

In a Zoom meeting, your boss would commend you for productivity, tripling your previous best performance.

Nobody knows you were on a manic episode last week, not even you.

In a Facebook marketplace, you exchanged three kilos of rice for a can of Spam, the little things that matter.

xxii. *Didn't they say it comes as a black dog-shaped smoke? To you, it comes as a hovering voice, a litany of sins.*

xxiii. Over Viber, you send a therapy meme from Twitter to your shrink. He replies that he's worried about you, asks if you thought about committing to the institution for a few weeks. You dread his incessant "How do you feel today?" queries. You loathe questions you don't have answers to. You crave certainty, the known.

Over Google Meet, he would look at you with intent like a school principal and say, "I've read your latest published piece…" he goes on, "I must say…" While you normally detest this form of surveillance—he obviously put your name on Google alert as you are a patient that needs constant monitoring—you view conversations like this way better.

xxiv. Twenty-One Pilots' "Level of Concern" has been on repeat on Spotify. Sing the part where Tyler Joseph repeatedly says, "Tell me we're alright, tell me we're okay." In your SMS inbox, three unread messages from two ex-friends and your father. Ex-friends had no idea you've cut them off. You call your father tonight, a first since 2018.

xxv. At least five submissions calling for literary response to the current events are in your newsfeed, as if more poetry can solve it all. ("But they help us make sense," a poet-friend would tell you.) A poet you idolize critiqued anthologies with natural and human-made disasters as impetus: "There is something amiss in collective action when all that comes out of it is more poetry." Decline the insistent invitations. Do not romanticize this kind of catharsis. But you failed in the *not romanticizing* part. You wrote a flash nonfiction triptych—or is it a prose poem suite? —about meeting a Tinder date who lives on the other side of the city. Separated by a police checkpoint and a bridge as if it was the 38th parallel, recount the scene as if it is from a Korean drama, savoring in it, even settling for the crumbs that memory allowed for the taking.

Tim Roach's 2021 book *Screen Love: Queer Intimacies in the Grindr Era* has explained this: "Screens nourish a utopian impulse: that dead thing between us—the barrier reminding me, consciously or not, that I am alone—makes me want to reach out all the more. Even the most noncommittal online come-ons, clearly born of boredom, betray an all-too-human desire for connection: a change to the current situation, a chance…"

So, the next week, decide not to see him again. Romance in this economy, to you, seems impractical.

xxvi. *Didn't they say it comes as a black dog-shaped smoke? To you, it comes as a hovering voice, a litany of sins.*

xxvii. You miss the view of the city you're in, its panorama, the skyline during the blue hour right outside your window. When Joan Didion wrote in *Blue Nights*, "I had been alone in the apartment," or in *The Year of Magical Thinking*, "I had been alone in the kitchen of that house, late twilight, early evening," you felt that. Now draw the dusty curtains after a little sneeze, and let the remaining light of sunset in.

Bio: Alton Melvar M Dapanas (they/them), a native of southern Philippines, is the author of *Towards a Theory on City Boys: Prose Poems* (UK: Newcomer Press, 2021), assistant non-fiction editor at London-based *Panorama: The Journal of Intelligent Travel*, Iowa-based *Atlas & Alice Literary Magazine*, and editorial reader at *Creative Nonfiction*. Published in Sweden, Lebanon, Germany, Nigeria, Taiwan, USA, Austria, Japan, and Netherlands, their latest works have appeared in *Modern Poetry in Translation* (UK), *Tolka Journal* (Ireland), *New Contrast* (South Africa), *The Best Asian Poetry* (Singapore), *Mekong Review* (Australia), *Canthius Magazine* (Canada), and *Poetry Lab Shanghai (China)* where they were translated into the Chinese.

MANIA AND DEPRESSION:

TWO SIDES OF THE SAME COIN

by Rae Shane

Mania and depression aren't all that different, really. While the term "bipolar" implies that they are two opposite sides of the spectrum, they're both mental states that produce thought errors, causing the inflicted to think and believe illogical and hyperbolic statements about themselves. The problem is that the person suffering has an extremely difficult time noticing the improbability of the thoughts – because we as a society are taught to identify with the mind so closely, those suffering from bipolar take on their minds' wild stories as if they were scientific evidence.

Both mania and depression cause the mind to tell stories so engrossing that they can become spirals and cycles of emotion. As someone diagnosed with bipolar in my late 20s, I had become very familiar with these narratives when I experienced my worst episodes. The apex of the saga came right before my diagnosis, and my experience with the two poles encapsulated the stories my brain had told me my entire life.

Depression told me I was the worst.

"I found this place in the Netherlands that euthanizes people with severe mental health issues," I said plainly during a therapy appointment while in the throes of the darkest depression of my life.

I used every rational argument I could think of to get a referral to the program: I was in excruciating pain daily. Tormenting thoughts swarmed my brain, mostly about how I should be dead and how worthless I was; I saw no way out of that. I had been battling depression on and off since age eight. I figured that's how it's always supposed to be, that it was part of my personality now. The medication and magnet treatment (TMS) I tried weren't improving things. I wanted to give my therapist and my mom the option to do things the easy way—pay someone to end my life clinically so I didn't have to do the dirty work myself.

I knew being referred would be a long shot, that I would be rebuffed. Although, in a suicidal state of mind, I truly believed that this was the right course of action. I felt that I had nothing left and I couldn't possibly see a future. When I tried, all I saw was complete darkness, as if I were endlessly falling through a hole in the ground. Anxious, obsessive-compulsive, and depressive thoughts raced rapidly through my mind relentlessly. My symptoms were not only mental; my physical health was completely shot. It was as if someone filled my limbs with wet cement; I could move them around, but they felt three times heavier than they normally were. Hot coals lined the space around my heart, so much so that a dull burning sensation lived in my chest for those four months I lived in excruciating pain.

My symptoms were so severe that I took time off work to tend to my condition, which my perfectionistic brain saw as a complete failure. I didn't see a world in which I could recover from that interruption in my career, which had already been disrupted by mental health issues in the past. In my depression, my second breakdown was "proof" that I would never be able to support myself again. I was so steeped in capitalistic brainwashing at the time that I completely wrapped up my worth in how productive I could be and how well my bosses and colleagues thought I was doing. I remembered the words my ex-colleague and friend gave me years before: "It's just a job." However, as much as I tried, I couldn't internalize that mantra. It was more than work to me. At the time, it was a key part of the narrow view of my identity.

None of the other factors of my perceived "purpose" were really panning out as I had hoped at the time. I felt consistently disconnected from my friends, like I was always on the fringe of my group. My depressive thoughts told me I was only included in activities or invited to things out of pity. On the relationship front, I had been dumped by many of the serious boyfriends I ever had, and I considered all of those personal failings. I assumed I was a terrible dog owner because I struggled to get out of bed and wasn't providing a positive environment for my pet. I figured I was a complete burden on my family because I was staying with them while I was on suicide watch. If all these identities were shattered, what did I have left? Where could I source any sense of pride?

Without an identity, I barely considered myself a human being. I'd contemplate how it would be if I jumped in front of a bullet train, thinking about how I could time it precisely, making it the least painful death. It was the only respite I got from a gut-wrenching existence—the idea that I could potentially escape. What people don't realize is that suicide isn't a choice; it's an incredibly dangerous symptom that most people—even mental health professionals—treat like a character flaw.

Despite the shame, guilt, and almost constant suicidal thoughts, I had split seconds of hope periodically. There was something in the back of my mind that urged, "Stay. See what happens." It was a quiet but confident command. Somehow, I decided to listen over and over.

Despite that nudge, it was still easy to ignore in the depths of my existential dread. However, as the medication started working, and when I finally got off the waitlist into a partial hospitalization program (PHP), I started to listen to that voice more often. That's when my life all started to turn around—at a snail's pace, but it did.

During the program, which lasted six hours every weekday for six weeks, I continued to feel isolated and alone—despite attending group sessions with a handful of others with depression. I assumed I was the most severe case and was the only person in the group who admitted to suicidal ideation on the daily intake sheet. Even though I felt painfully alone, those tiny spots of hope crept into my day-to-day more often. "Stay. Fulfill your purpose," said the voice. I named her Gladys. I was committed to getting out of this, if not for me, then for Gladys.

Each day, I made a Herculean effort to try and see a future, even if I was just making microscopal progress. I slowly started to realize that I was not my job title, that my family didn't see me as a burden, and that I could see myself as valuable. When I finally started to see the possibility of escaping my nightmare, I began researching articles on reasons why I should stay alive. Surprisingly, I didn't find any practical tips on how to stop feeling suicidal in those "don't kill yourself" essays online. They told me cliches, such as, "Think about the stuff you liked to do before you were depressed," and, "Think about how you'd affect your loved ones if you killed yourself." There were no words of encouragement out there that gave me the will to continue enduring constant physical and mental anguish. I only found what worked for me when I started combining my own unconventional ideas with therapy strategies. That's when I started to take back the narrative. Unfortunately, that more positive story turned into my first full-blown manic and psychotic episode.

Mania told me I was the best.

I never really considered myself as someone with a life calling until, one day, I woke up and thought, "I'm going to save the world—as a porn star."

Historically, I was never one to be so public about my sexuality, so it was a confusing surprise to my family and friends when I started posting things like, "$4,000 FOR PUSSY PICS!" on Facebook. In just a few days, I had gotten requests for hundreds of new social media friends, who I assumed were "leads" for my entrepreneurial porn business. I didn't get why my loved ones couldn't understand my marketing tactics, and I continued full force.

Hypersexuality is often a key part of manic episodes. At the time, I had no idea—it was my first experience with an episode that severe. Even more terrifying was that my first bout of mania included elements of psychosis, which came with extreme delusions. Throughout the process, I believed that I was fated to be a famous porn star named Cherry who would save the world by spreading unadulterated, communal love in all her films. In my exploding mind, Cherry was destined to make the skeptics believe in love again through the guise of sexuality. Now, that's a comic book I want to read, but not a reality I want to live. Don't get me wrong, I believe sex work is legitimate and should be legalized for a number of reasons. However, when hypersexuality is uncharacteristic of someone and they're exhibiting it in such an overt way, it's a symptom.

In the thick of it, Cherry was on a divine quest from the Universe, and I would stop at nothing to fulfill my humanity-saving quest. When my mom showed up unannounced at my apartment to stop me from my manic mission, I lashed out, feeling suffocated by her presence. She understandably expressed her concern for the explicit content I was sharing with nearly everyone I knew. To her horror, I fell into a fit of giggles; I guess this is the most appropriate time to say that I was laughing maniacally. I have to say, my mom deserves an Oscar for that interaction. She played it extremely cool for the mother of a girl who lost her mind. In hindsight, I could tell she had pored over articles and books about how to interact with someone in the throes of this disordered state. Not many people could have kept their cool in that way.

In one instance, I was sitting on my bed, texting people incomprehensible messages in a rapid-fire way. I told friends their fortunes, convinced I was an all-knowing and a powerful psychic. The way I spoke about these abilities indicated that I was experiencing delusions of grandeur, another manic symptom. In a group text, I predicted that my girlfriends were all about to become rich simply because they were associated with me. I pushed the idea onto my friend that she would be my manager when I became a famous public figure.

I then glanced up from my phone, where I saw my mom on my couch, quietly on her phone. For some reason, that made me seethe with anger. As if someone pressed the "self-destruct" button on me, I *had* to get out of the apartment. At that moment, my mom was the enemy. She was keeping me from my ultimate destination of fame. I couldn't stand her presence, as if she was a stinking cockroach that I couldn't squash, so I had to flee the site. I told her I needed to get the mail then sprinted down the block in the early morning hours, the streets still dark.

Just a quick thirty seconds later, a man in grey clothing next to a white van called me over to him. I walked over with the confidence and sultriness of Dita Von Teese, staring him fearlessly in the eyes as I proceeded to tell him I was going to be a famous porn star. He offered to drive me to Los Angeles to start my journey, so of course Cherry agreed wholeheartedly. He turned to me ominously, and he mentioned that he needed to make sure I was ready. With that, the man grabbed my ass with both hands as I disassociated, like it was just an annoying part of my future job. When he deemed my rear worthy, he opened the car door for me. I grabbed at the seatbelt automatically, and he looked disapprovingly at me.

"No seatbelts," he scolded.

"Oh, right," I said, acting as if I knew the reasoning behind it. One of my symptoms was feeling invincible—a common idea in mania—so I assumed that it was to prove how truly indestructible we were. I thought he was like me – all-powerful in our mission to fulfill our purposes together.

"We need to check to see if you can be a *really* great porn star," he started.

I boldly challenged him, saying, "Go ahead, test me." With that, he slapped me as hard as he could across my face.

"How was that?" he asked.

"Fine. I didn't feel a thing," I said nonchalantly. I truly didn't feel pain as strongly as I would have in a less activated brain state.

"Oh, really?" he asked. He struck me even harder. This time, my eyes welled up with tears.

"Totally fine."

In that moment, it was almost as if the blow across my face gave me a glimpse of my old self. In a flash, I saw my family in my mind's eye, wondering what they would think if they knew a stranger was assaulting me. I started feeling the collective pain of people who had been physically abused. A hint of empathy and regret creeped back into my psyche.

"Let's check out this beach," the man suggested. With that, I snapped right back to psychosis, thinking this natural setting would bring me a sign of where I should start with Cherry's career.

Time was warped while I was manic and psychotic. One moment, I was laughing and playing alone on the beach as the man fiddled on his phone. The next thing I knew, I was in a strange town, hours away. He took my ID and abandoned me in a parking lot. In my overconfident cloud, I wasn't worried about it at all. I figured I'd get to LA to start my career somehow, and I was very occupied when I found a tiny grey stray cat in a tree.

I had this feeling that it was the reincarnated spirit of my late grandmother, so I was determined to wait until that cat came down to be with me. While I believe in some form of reincarnation when I'm in my right mind, magical thinking in this extreme is another symptom of psychosis. I was fully wrapped up in the grips of my severe symptoms.

Somehow, in this dream-like scenario, I came around to a lightbulb moment – my mom was actually trying to help me in my expedition to become Cherry the porn star! Somewhere in my chaotic, racing thoughts, I figured that I had been wrong about her all along. In a frenzy, I asked a stranger with a trim mustache in a RAV4 if I could use his phone, and I called my mom to see if she could come get me.

My parents acted quickly when they heard from me. My dad contacted a friend of a friend who was a firefighter in the town, who showed up calmly and amicably to make sure I stayed safe until my mother arrived. Time became fuzzy again, and the next thing I knew, I was at a hospital in San Francisco, telling other patients' fortunes by interpreting playing cards. Finally, I was able to gradually come down from the high. Then the crash came back.

***

Both mania and depression are destructive, keeping those with the illness under its spell; as the Earth keeps turning, the sufferer's world often stops. That makes it easy to fall into the trap of thinking, "I'm different than everyone else," either in a positive or negative way. The antidote for me? Remembering my place in the human ecosystem – while we all have unique traits, I'm really not so different than anyone else. I now have the space from my thoughts to realize that I am part of the human ecosystem, just like anyone else. I'm no better nor worse than anyone. In fact, there is no such thing as objective better or worse, and that keeps me grounded in my stable brain state.

Bio: Rae Shane is a passionate mental health advocate and enjoys volunteering with a national mental illness advocacy organization. During the week, she works in the technology field in San Francisco. Aside from her volunteer and day jobs, Rae enjoys hanging out with her terrier and loves discovering new psychology podcasts.

FINDING SUNSHINE

by Kelly Esparza

Sometimes I feel as if I'm a prisoner in my own mind and body. Sometimes I feel as if I'm speaking to the world behind glass. Detached. Disconnected. Sometimes my mind feels like a tornado, self-destructive and dangerous. I get lost in the twists and the turns, the labyrinth of my overthinking mind. Anxiety makes my thoughts restless and loud; in contrast, depression belittles and silences me. Other times, depression convinces me of the opposite of what I think and clouds my overall thinking and behavior. I'm a stormy day, even when there isn't anything wrong, even when my day should be sunny.

Mental ill-health is still stigmatized. Sure, there's the "it's okay not to be okay" movement on social media, but mental health isn't normalized like it should be. "How are you?" A simple, polite question we ask each other daily. The typical response is, "I'm good. How are you?" It's expected from society to say you're doing well, even when you're not. I can fall into this trap, giving in to the expectation, the norm. And sometimes I feel like a liar because I'm not always "well" when I'm asked, but saying, "I'm good" rolls off my tongue, like it's the most natural thing to say.

Unfortunately, talking about mental health still isn't as accepted as it needs to be. Why? I believe it's the fear of being judged, of being seen as weak, of being rejected by others. And sadly, some people choose to judge and to reject, but we must remember that not everyone will. But that still leads into the ultimate fear of *always* being rejected for how we feel, think, act. And it's that fear in which sometimes I feel like a computer glitch, except that's where I'm wrong. We aren't computers; we're human beings. Human beings with the ability to feel emotions. We aren't meant to be perfect. I used to think I felt too much, and maybe sometimes I still think that way. But mental ill-health is a part of us, what we deal with, what we must learn to cope with. What I have learned, however, is that it doesn't define us.

It doesn't take a rocket scientist to figure out I've always dealt with anxiety. From a young age, I knew that, on some level, I always felt more anxious than the average person. It was the little things, like worrying about being late, anticipation for the first day of school, test anxiety, or handling change in general. However, at the time, I didn't realize anxiety could be an actual disorder.

I had my first panic attack in high school. It was terrible and unlike anything I had ever experienced before. It was my sophomore year, and I was taking a test in my honors chemistry class. An overwhelming fear attacked me unexpectedly. My breath caught in my throat. My chest felt heavy, like an elephant sat there, and instinctively, my hand reached up, my fingertips massaging my heart that was beating fast—too fast. In my mind, my messy, overthinking thoughts are always like a bunch of entangled knots, but in that instant, my thoughts were no longer cluttered but blank. My mouth and throat instantly felt as dry as the Arizona desert, and my fingertips grew numb and tingly. I felt frozen in place. When I later spoke to my chemistry teacher, I found out she used to experience this exact same sensation, which was a panic attack. I'd never heard of the term before, nor had I ever experienced one. Unfortunately, this was only the beginning of many more panic attacks to come.

I remember crying once in an English class because I had this same overwhelming anxiety. As it was like when I was younger, it was always the little things that caused my generalized anxiety and panic attacks. I was in a seminar, discussing a book I'd read and analyzed. The class sat in a large circle. My notes were scattered on my desk, and I bent my head, looking down, avoiding eye contact with my teacher. I was never one to like speaking up in class; for some reason, my heart sped up, and my hands even became clammy just thinking of the idea. I'd always paid attention; the fear of speaking in a big group, though, was enough to make my heartbeat compete with the sounds of each of the students speaking. Despite my efforts, my teacher called on me to share my thoughts, and I froze, just as I had that day when I took my chemistry test. I remember the eyes of the students focusing on me, listening intently, waiting for me to speak. Except I couldn't. My cheeks burned like fire, I became breathless, as if I'd stood up too quickly, dizzy, and I stammered, my mind once again going blank. Before I knew it—or could even stop it—tears streamed down my cheeks, creating a small puddle on my desk.

To say I was embarrassed would be an understatement. I was *mortified*. I knew crying wasn't anything to be ashamed of, but nevertheless, I wasn't a fan of crying in front of others. At that moment, I was trembling from that intense panic attack. My teacher pulled me aside after class to ask if I was okay, and at the time, I said yes because all I wanted was to get out of there as quickly as possible. And I probably was calm by the time the panic attack ended, but in retrospect, was I really okay? No. I didn't fully understand how to cope with anxiety at the time, and unfortunately, this wouldn't be the only time I'd cry from a panic attack in public.

Depression is never that far behind anxiety. It pulls me under its current like a tidal wave, and every time I think I've thrashed to the surface, feeling better, feeling like my old self again, another depressive episode pulls me back under. Depression is the definition of what it means to emotionally drown. A heaviness cloaks you, weighs you down until it's even difficult to find the strength to do simple tasks, such as getting out of bed in the morning, eating, or taking a shower. Whispers of self-doubt, self-critique, and negativity creep into your mind until they gradually become louder, transitioning into screams that you were once able to turn around into positive thoughts but are now unable to. Depression is like poison; it starts in your mind, spreading quickly throughout your body until it reaches your heart, and you feel as if you lose the spark that makes you, *you* for a while.

It wasn't until my senior year of high school that I was officially diagnosed with anxiety and depression. For me, anxiety was all consuming when it happened, and it's now that I think depression is like anxiety's shadow, lingering until eventually depression in itself takes over, like a solar eclipse. Together, they feel suffocatingly unstoppable, like a team of supervillains seeking power. What makes mental ill-health difficult is that sometimes you know you need help, but you don't know how to go about it. You want someone to wave a magic wand over you, causing every trace of your depression and anxiety to disappear, but the fact is, there isn't a quick fix to either of these, no matter how much you wish there was.

When thinking about mental health, I think society doesn't know how to normalize it in some ways. Therapists always say that having a friend or a family member to talk to is a healthy way to cope with anxiety and depression, but what if that loved one doesn't know what to say or how to comfort you when you need someone the most, especially if they don't know what depression or anxiety feels like? Why isn't there more literature that discusses mental health for all ages? Why don't we see this in film more often? Why isn't mental health more accurately represented?

Now time and time again, I've had therapists tell me to get a journal and to write my thoughts down. I've tried this on numerous occasions without any success. It can be helpful for some, I suppose, to keep a journal, hand writing your deepest thoughts, sorrows, frustrations, reflections of gratitude. But this never works for me, no matter how hard I try. However, it's times like these that society needs to remember that there isn't one correct way to cope.

Creative writing has always been an outlet for me in times of stress. It's where I'm happiest, where I can let my mind wander, where I can be lost in another imaginative world that I create. As a novelist, I often connect this with the fact that I run long distances when I'm anxious or depressed. Both can be challenging in terms of length and stamina to finish strong, while also being equally as rewarding in the long term. Depression and anxiety make you feel weak, physically, mentally, and emotionally, even though you know deep down you aren't. The dedication, determination, and accomplishment when it comes to finishing writing a novel or running a 5k race helps me to see that I am mentally and physically strong, even when I feel as if I'm not. Both outlets challenge me to fight, to push back against depression's tidal waves and anxiety's unexpected attacks from behind.

During my freshman year of college, I had a few depressive episodes. I recall being on edge, anxious more days than I wasn't. I cried often. Moving to a new state for college was challenging. Discovering a balance and a routine were difficult. That summer after my freshman year, I debated going back or transferring, but I decided to try one more year. I began reading *Wild* by Cheryl Strayed. Her self-discovery memoir inspired me to push through what I felt at the time, to not give up despite the pain I felt from depression and anxiety. This was also when running saved my life. As a former soccer and track athlete, I wasn't a stranger to running. I started from the beginning—from being completely out of shape—to getting where I wanted to be. I transitioned from middle distance running to long distance. It wasn't easy, but neither was coping with panic attacks and depression. The repetition, the constant determination to improve, and the release of endorphins helped my mental health immensely. I trained and entered myself in 5k races for the first time, working to beat my own personal best times at each race, which I did successfully. When it comes to anxiety and depression, both can be equally isolating and make you feel empty on the inside. In contrast, running can be a solitary activity, but one that helps me to work through the emotional pain. While it's important to seek help with mental health if needed, coping with anxiety and depression are still personal battles; I see running the same way. Running in the rain, against the wind, in the blazing heat, uphill—each scene is a battle that I personally strive to overcome. Ultimately, I feel as powerful as a superhero when I run and push myself to face my fears up front.

Writing poetry has also become an active outlet for me to express and to process anything I felt. In this way, poetry became my journaling, as I realized journaling can take many forms. I just needed to find an activity that better suited my needs, that came naturally to me and was cathartic, that worked for me so that I could express myself. At first, my poetry was dark and somber, detailing my depressive episodes, but this has changed in recent years. Along with writing poetry, I started reading it more, consuming poets' words, healing from the pressure I consistently placed on myself. It was then that I noticed a majority of the collections I read focused solely on the depressive state of mind, which is helpful to relate to, but at the same time, I hardly read any poetry that answered the "so then what happened" question. I didn't find much poetry that demonstrated fighting against depression and anxiety and breaking free from them with the help of inner strength, loved ones, and positive thoughts.

Ultimately, it was then that my writing shifted. Although my poems would begin sadly, they would end on a positive note, focusing on finding one's own peace, strength, and love from within. I figured if I wanted others to read my work, I wanted them to feel happier and hopeful and potentially inspired that they could rise above the mental, physical, and emotional challenges they face. Poetry became my go-to when I was depressed, anxious, or overall upset.

Now, I wish I could say that my depression and anxiety are gone forever because of the activities I've discovered that help me, but I can't. There are months I feel unstoppable and happy as can be. And then other times, everything comes crashing down, and I must rebuild again. Mental health is about being aware, mindful, and taking action to find a balance, to discover what helps you to shine.

Depression and anxiety slammed into me whenever I least expected it—like with the pandemic. Although I'd like to say I've accomplished a lot even with these difficult times, both proved to be challenging. While I knew other emotions could mask themselves as depression and anxiety, I don't think I completely knew to what extent. From the chaos of uncertainty, to finishing my last semester of college, to moving home and looking for a job all amidst a pandemic, anxiety placed me on a rollercoaster ride, sliding me right, left, up, down, making me dizzy from the impact. Depression, like it does, slinked behind, waiting, daring to emerge and to bite like a snake when my anxiety subsided.

Depression became a shapeshifter, manifesting itself as a recurring nightmare, in episodes of insomnia, anger and irritability, physical aches that latched onto my body, emotional numbness, and definitive decisions I struggled to make. Once again, I became a storm on a supposed-to-be sunny day, feeling hopeless and unworthy once more. But like every time, I learned how to swim, and I didn't let myself drown under the pressure. I found a routine during the pandemic, incorporating a schedule to keep me busy and productive. Just like the little anxieties I felt, there were little rays of sunshine I found to turn myself around for the better.

Yoga and meditation became daily habits, helping to place my anxiety to rest, lifting my mood when I felt down. I strove to run outside every other day, getting sunshine, working through my stresses in a familiar way. I set goals for myself, running farther until I ran three, four, five miles or more without struggling, writing a little each day, spending time with my family and friends, finding projects that gave me purpose and motivation to keep moving forward. When depression hits, it's difficult to find joy, to carry on with what makes me, *me*, but sometimes focusing on placing one foot in front of the other is what pushes me to find myself once more.

Depression and anxiety are a part of what I deal with, but they don't define me. Although I wish I could say I won't have to cope with them in the future, I know I will, but I'd like to think that the harder I fight back, the stronger I become, even when I don't feel like it, and it takes me a moment to believe that I'm strong once more. With the help of those around me and the activities that make me feel empowered, I know that I'll break free from depression and anxiety's captivity, and I'll always find my sunshine again.

Bio: Kelly Esparza is a California-based editor and writer who holds a B.A. in English and a B.A. in Creative Writing from the University of Arizona. Her personal essays, short stories, and poetry have appeared in various literary journals and anthologies. In early 2021, she co-wrote a screenplay for a feature film, and her published short story, "Destiny Says" (*Analogies and Allegories Literary Magazine*, 2021), received a Pushcart Prize nomination. Find out more on her website: kellyesparza.wordpress.com. Her Twitter is @Kelly_Esparza7.

HIS NAME WAS JOSH

by Trisha Martin

I choke down a gulp of coffee that has long since gone cold as I gently type thoughtful words to a mother who is beside herself with grief. She lost her daughter two months ago and is looking for comfort in others who have experienced a similar loss. Visiting these forums each morning is the norm for me now. Yesterday it was a teen who lost his sister, and, the day before that, it was a grandmother who lost her grandson. I see hundreds of posts like these every day, and though our stories are vastly different, we are connected by a single, undeniable thread – suicide. Sometimes I am able to offer some reassurance to people who are going down a path I have already trudged. There are no words I can say to make the situation better, yet there is solace in knowing we are not alone. As I finish my response and click send, it dawns on me; I have a lifetime membership to a club no one wants to be a part of. I didn't ask to join and yet I can never get out.

On a daily basis, there are sights, sounds, and smells that trigger memories of my brother. Sometimes grief is subtle, other times it crashes down on you with unrelenting intensity. You learn to live with that heaviness; it's almost as if it becomes a part of you. The only consistent part of grief is that it is always present. Josh was three years older than me and I always looked up to him. He was handsome and athletic; I was quirky and clumsy. We had the same light eyes and we both had a tendency to laugh at things that weren't supposed to be funny. Josh had a wonderful bellowing laugh. I miss that a lot. There were times we would laugh until we couldn't breathe at jokes no one else understood. We made a great team. Josh was impulsive and fearless whereas I was more reserved and thoughtful. His spontaneity was something I always admired, and he often looked to me for insight. Josh and I definitely butted heads when we were younger, and even in adulthood we would often disagree, but we balanced each other. In him I had such security to be who I was. He let me tag along with his friends and he always kept a protective eye over me. He truly was an amazing big brother. In his absence, I've had to rediscover myself.

I can still vividly remember the look on Josh's face when he and our Dad presented me with my first bike. They had fixed up an old bicycle with pink spray paint, new white tires, and tiny training wheels. Dad placed a purple helmet on my head and pulled the strap under my chin so tight I felt like my chubby cheeks might explode. That is one of my favorite childhood memories. Just like that, Josh and I were off. Josh was faster and stronger, but he slowed down for me, gracing me with a patience that most people wouldn't believe he had. Josh had ADHD and sometimes struggled to focus, but he never faltered to give me his full attention. It wasn't long before he convinced me to ditch the training wheels; only moments later my false sense of confidence lifted as my knee collided with the pavement. Josh laughed a little before helping me up. I got back on my bike and tried again. Josh smiled and cheered at my resilience; he was my biggest fan and I always wanted to impress him.

Our father was a soldier, and during this time, we were living on an Army base in Alaska. The streets were dotted with small, uniform townhomes. It was the perfect spot to play, except for one grouchy dog a few houses down. The dog's owners kept him tethered, so we never worried too much about it. One day we were out riding our bikes and, as we sped around the curve of the sidewalk, Josh stopped to pick up a coin on the cement. As he placed it in his pocket, I whizzed past him taking full advantage of the opportunity to beat him home. We were not actually racing, but as the younger sibling, any opportunity where I was in the lead became a race. As I whizzed down the sidewalk, I caught a glimpse of the snarling dog in the corner of my eye. Common sense would have been to slow down and veer off the sidewalk a bit to avoid the dog, but I wanted to beat Josh home. Turns out, the dog had a new chain, and it was just a touch longer. The dog was now able to reach the sidewalk. After months of being taunted by our spinning wheels, he finally had his opportunity. He lunged at me, grabbing my back tire. As the dog pulled my bike from under me, my body smashed against the ground, and the dog's teeth dug into my hip. It was then that the panic set in and I let out an overly dramatic scream. In true big-brother fashion Josh came speeding to my rescue. He jumped off his bike and a sound somewhere between a yodel and a war cry filled the air. Josh had spent eight years watching Ninja Turtles and had unknowingly been trained for this exact moment. His lanky legs carried him briskly towards me. In one strong leap he flew through the air like a ninja, planting his foot on the dog's rump with a "Hi-YAW!" Startled, the dog retreated. Josh used all of his might to drag me home. When we walked through the front door of our home, Josh must have felt 100 feet tall. I explained to our mother how he had saved me. Looking back, I am fairly certain the dog just hated bike tires; the bite didn't leave me with any more than a bruised rear and a fear of dogs. Nonetheless, Josh was there when I needed him.

My family left Alaska the following year when my father retired from the military. We moved several times over the years before settling down in my parents' hometown in Texas. I was in elementary school when the beast my dad had been fighting began to surface. He was experiencing PTSD and depression related to some experiences from his time in the Army. Due to this, most of my childhood memories center around Josh and my mother. I always felt my parents took good care of us. We were happy, healthy kids. Through the years Josh and I fell into a steady groove; I was the whiney little sister and he was the pestering older brother. We played our roles faithfully. When I entered my freshman year of high school, Josh entered his first year at college. It was the first time in my life to not have him as a constant presence. College seemed awesome and I felt special knowing he took time out of a busy schedule to call and see how I was doing. During this time, our father was having a difficult time with his own mental health and our mother was doing her best to maintain a family business, be present for me, and take care of Dad. My mother has always had a beautiful knack for balancing life. Josh was a pillar of strength for me during that time. He reminded me to be patient with Dad and encouraged me to help Mom out whenever I could. He even ditched a date once to come home and console me after a break-up. His words were, "That guy sucked anyway. You will do better."

I guess that missed date did not matter much in the long run for Josh. I was a freshman in college when Josh met the woman who would later become his wife and the mother to his children. Stephanie was fun to be around and she quickly became a member of our family. Together they built a life they loved and welcomed two healthy children into this world. In 2012, when Josh's youngest child was only three months old, our family was thrown a curveball – Josh was sick. It started with stomach pains and escalated quickly to severe gastrointestinal distress. One day, when the symptoms were at their worst, he went to the ER. The on-call doctor ordered x-rays of his stomach. The x-ray tech was young and inexperienced. He accidentally took the first images too high. That accident is how we found out that my brother had been living with a life-threatening condition. He was born with congenital diaphragmatic hernia that had steadily grown over the years. The doctor informed us this condition is typically treated in infancy, but had been missed somehow. He compared the pressure on Josh's organs to a walking time bomb. Additional scans revealed his intestines were not only in his chest cavity but fused to segments of his heart and lungs. His insides were literally suffocating him. My brother needed surgery immediately or he would die.

The surgeon had to remove a large portion of Josh's intestines as well as a section of his left lung. The operation felt like it took decades. When it was finally over, I was taken to see him. The air of the surgical ICU felt cold and stale. Constant beeping echoed down the halls. Josh was hooked to so many tubes and wires, he was almost unrecognizable. When he saw me, he forced a little smile, trying once again to assure me everything would be okay. I was not so sure. I had never seen someone in such intense physical pain. I prayed without ceasing for God to heal him. His recovery was brutal. He was left with nerve damage, which caused intense and unrelenting pain. I thought we had overcome the worst, but he never truly recovered from that surgery. Over time, Josh became dependent on pain medication and began to lose interest in things that had once brought him joy. At one point following his surgery, Josh reached out to his care team about his increasing anxiety and depression. They told him that, given the ordeal he had experienced, his feelings were "normal and expected." He was not offered any treatment or advice. It was a long time before he spoke out about his mental health again. I can't help but wonder how often mental illness is dismissed in its earliest days when it is most treatable. How many other lives have been ruined by a lack of mental health awareness?

In the years following Josh's surgery, my husband and I moved off and started our own family. Life was chaotic and I did not do a good enough job staying in contact with my brother. We texted regularly, but he never opened up about how much he was struggling. The details that ultimately led to Josh's death are not mine to tell, and in all honesty, I will never know the exact sequence of events that initiated my brother's downward spiral. The gist of the story, to the best of my knowledge, is that at some point drugs and mental illness worked together to create the perfect storm for destroying the life my brother had worked so hard to build. He turned to drugs out of desperation after being dismissed by the medical professionals who were supposed to be his advocates. His wife left him, not because she did not love him, but because she genuinely couldn't handle the situation any longer. His children came to live with my parents. Even at his worst, Josh made it a point to make sure his children were safe and he felt that was their best option. We all thought it was temporary. We expected Josh and Stephanie to work things out, and both get the medical care they needed, but weeks turned to months and months turned to years. Truthfully, by the time we realized Josh needed professional help, he was already in a really bad spot mentally. Josh saw numerous medical professionals and even had some time inpatient at mental health facilities, but I don't think he was ever fully open with anyone due to distrust. He always felt doctors were not truly on his side. He felt like he was viewed as a burden. The reality is it was easier for my brother to have access to methamphetamines and marijuana than it was for him to see a psychiatrist. It takes a lot of inner strength for someone who is struggling with mental health to seek help, and our system demands that they find the strength to do it not once, but repeatedly. We don't make cancer patients beg for chemo, so why do we wait for mental health patients to have mental breakdowns before recognizing the severity of their disease?

Little by little my own brother became someone I hardly knew. It felt like I lost two of my best friends because both Josh and Stephanie had changed so much. I always clung to hope that things would get better. I viewed the whole situation as a rough patch, truly believing it was temporary. I made it a point to be present in my niece and nephew's lives from the very beginning. When things got rough with their parents, I was consistent. I know Josh really appreciated that. Josh was no longer the fun loving, kind man I had known. He became unpredictable and distant. We had once been able to talk endlessly and openly about everything, but in the last couple of years before his death even simple conversations were challenging. Sometimes we got glimpses of the man he used to be, but those moments had become sparse. We pleaded so intensely with him to get more help, to the point that he began to shut us out. I wish I had never stopped pushing. My only sibling never got the chance to truly be an uncle to my children. Josh could have been the best dad and best uncle in the whole world and he wanted to. Mental illness robbed us of that. Mental illness stole my brother from me and left me with a broken heart and a lifetime of unfinished plans.

People always want to know how it happened, and while I do know the details of how Josh died, I still do not understand it. The day my brother ended his life started off wonderfully and ended with more shock and horror than I knew possible. I had come into town to visit my family for the first time since the COVID-19 pandemic broke out. I talked to Josh that morning and we laughed about how his dog looked like Master Splinters, the rat from Ninja Turtles. It was a nice day in mid-May, so the kids were in the backyard swimming. Mom and I stepped in to start preparing an afternoon snack while enjoying the kid's joyful squeals. Josh and Dad were out running errands and were expected to be home soon. I mentioned to Mom that they should have been back by now. She nodded in agreement and grabbed her phone. Suddenly, the ring of my mother's phone pierced the air with an intensity that shocked me. As soon as she answered it, the color left her face. The tone of my mother's voice and the terror in her eyes replay in my memory. I stood back in silence as I overheard a conversation that is now burned into my mind's eye with an unrelenting permanence. My mother choked out the words, "Is he dead?!" My father went silent. He couldn't say the words. A police officer came on the line and gave his condolences.

My brother died at 33 years old from a self-inflicted gunshot wound. His children were only eight and ten years old, and we had to tell them what had happened. How do you help a child understand a loss you don't understand yourself? I suppose grace is the only answer there. Later, the police officer told us Josh had called his mental health clinic three times that morning. They didn't return his call. I wonder what he would have said to them. Was he going to ask for help? Why didn't he say anything to us? I will never have those answers. Josh's cause of death was ruled "Suicide: gunshot wound," but we know the bullet is not what really took my brother from us, mental illness did.

I now realize my brother's story is just one of many. Suicide loss is far more common than most realize. Symptoms of mental illness, such as depression and psychosis, can vary from individual to individual and they can mimic numerous other medical conditions. Additionally, it is not uncommon for people experiencing complex mental illness to attempt to self-medicate with drugs or alcohol, making diagnosis and treatment even more challenging. In all honesty, I thought my brother was still using drugs though he had assured me he was clean. I was devastated when his toxicology report from the autopsy confirmed there were no substances in his system because I knew I had made a fatal mistake. My family mistook psychosis for drug use. They can look very similar and sometimes drugs can even induce psychosis. I know now psychosis is a medical emergency and should be treated as such. Signs to look for include increased difficulty concentrating, depressed or altered mood, sleeping too much or too little, anxiety, paranoia or suspicion, withdrawal from family and friends, delusional thinking, hallucinations, disorganized speech such as switching topics erratically, depression and suicidal thoughts or actions, or any abrupt change in personality. It is important to know that an individual is capable of being in psychosis and still seeming somewhat rational. That is what really threw us off and why Josh's doctors missed it. He knew what to say to them because he had a degree in psychology. We saw many of these symptoms in my brother but we failed to recognize the severity. Unfortunately, our medical system demands mentally ill individuals to be their own advocates if they are over 18 years of age. Most are simply unable. Each bout of psychosis makes additional bouts more likely. Josh spent the last years of his life going in and out of psychosis, and we were oblivious to the gravity of his struggles. He suffered immensely as he struggled to distinguish between reality and delusion. I imagine it must have been so scary. An early and proper diagnosis could have potentially changed the outcome of my brother's life. That is precisely why mental health awareness is so critical; lives are on the line.

After my brother's death, we did our best to pick up our lives and maintain normalcy for the kids, but nothing will ever be "normal" again. The pain my mother has experienced since losing her son is something so deep and primal that no words could ever bring justice to the level of heartache she endures daily. My father witnessed the incident and I cannot even begin to imagine how that affects him. When someone dies from cancer, a car accident, or a heart attack, people talk about who they were and the life they lived. Those conversations of remembrance help to bring forth healing. When someone dies by suicide, people talk about how they died, not who they were. I don't want my brother's death to outshine his life. That one moment of mental instability is not more important than the thousands of good moments that came before. My brother died by suicide, but he lived before he died.

Josh was funny, smart, and kind. Josh loved hard and fully. He was always there when someone needed him. He is missed daily by family and friends who were lucky enough to know the real him. Josh's death has been the most agonizing experience I have ever endured, but it has also made me a better person. I am more aware, more empathetic, and more thankful. Josh's absence is a constant reminder to me of the fragility of life. I want others to know it is okay to talk about mental illness and suicide. I know those conversations are uncomfortable, but open communication is the first step in dissipating the vicious stigma surrounding mental illness that plagues our society and prevents so many from seeking proper mental health treatment. If you or someone you care about is experiencing depression, anxiety, or any other symptom of mental illness, please reach out to those around you. Don't give up. "Too late" often comes faster than we realize.

Bio: Trisha Martin is a 32-year-old mother and homemaker. On May, 13, 2020, she lost her only sibling to suicide. This essay was written in his memory and depicts the struggles mental illness and suicide can produce.

REDEEMING JUDAS:

MEN, SUICIDE, AND HOPE

by Joe Haward

In Dante's *Inferno* we encounter the one who Virgil calls "Dis," the "Emperor of the sorrowful realm" who is also known as Satan. Dante describes Satan having "three faces in his head," a heretical inversion of the Christian Trinity, a picture invoking mockery towards who God is. From each mouth, tears and blood drip down as Satan tortures three people by holding them in his mouth, devouring them with his fangs, and flaying them with his claws. Virgil tells Dante to look up at the head of Satan, at the face in the middle where the greatest pain is being inflicted,

> "That wretch up there whom keenest pangs divide
> Is Judas called Iscariot," said my lord,
> "His head within, his jerking legs outside."[1]

Here in the ninth circle of Hell the worst of sinners reside, a place of fear, misery, and utter ruin. It is of no surprise that Dante locates Judas within this place, a place reserved for traitors and betrayers, or the "son of perdition," (John 17:12) as the New Testament puts it. His eternal destruction in Hell is described by Dante in the most horrific of ways, but fleetingly and almost as a passing comment. And, in the same way, his destruction in life is described with equal brevity by the writers

1 Dante, *The Divine Comedy*, Canto XXXIV.61

of the New Testament. The book of Acts puts these words in Peter's mouth about Judas,

> "Men, brothers, it was necessary that the scripture be fulfilled, which the Spirit, the Holy one, spoke beforehand through the mouth of David concerning Judas, who became a guide for those who arrested Jesus—For he was numbered among us, and had a share in this ministry—So that from the reward for his injustice this man purchased a field and, having fallen prone in the middle of it, he burst apart and all his entrails were poured out..." (Acts 1:16–18)

In the book of Matthew, the death of Judas is recorded like this,

> "Then Judas, the one who betrayed him, seeing that he had been condemned, changed his heart and returned the thirty silver pieces to the chief priests and elders, Saying, "I sinned by betraying innocent blood." But they said, "What is it to us? You will see to it." And flinging the silver pieces into the sanctuary he withdrew, and going away he hanged himself." (Matt 27:3–5)

A bronze plate from the doors of the Benevento Cathedral in Italy combines both these accounts of the death of Judas and show him hanging from a tree with his bowels hanging out. He is held by a Harpy, a winged creature from Greek mythology that were the spirits of sudden, strong gusts of wind that snatched people away, sometimes a creature that was associated with the underworld. Within Dante's world, Harpies were "wide-winged," "lady-faced," with "claws of steel." These Harpies dwell in the Seventh Circle of Hell, in the second ring where the Wood of the Suicides is found. Harpies sit on the branches of the trees where the souls of the damned are now entombed. Dante speaks of these trees in this way,

"No green here, but discolored leaves and dark,
No tender shoots, but written and gnarled and tough,
No fruit, but poison-galls on the withered bark."[1]

Dante snaps off a branch and the tree cries out in pain, with blood that flows from the broken branch.

"Why does thou rend my bones?"[2] the tree cries out.

He goes on,

"We that are turned to trees were human once;
Nay, thou shouldest tender a more pious hand
Though we had been the souls of scorpions."[3]

The Harpies sit on the branches, feeding on the leaves and biting the branches, providing agony to the souls of the suicides. It is little surprise, then, that the picture of the hanged Judas at Benevento Cathedral has a Harpy ready to carry Judas away.

The earliest known depiction of Christ's crucifixion in narrative form is from a small ivory carving, dated in the early part of the fifth century, with Judas hanging from a tree, his face upturned to the branch that suspends him, a bag of silver pieces at his feet.

The theologian, Karl Barth, (1886 – 1968) commenting on the death of Judas, puts it like this,

> ". . . Judas perished from within himself . . . His creaturely being could no longer endure the monstrousness of the contradiction in which he had enmeshed himself, and so it had to explode like a released hand-grenade."[4]

1 Dante, *The Divine Comedy*, Canto XIII.4
2 Dante, *The Divine Comedy*, Canto XIII.31
3 Dante, *The Divine Comedy*, Canto XIII.37
4 Karl Barth, *CD* II.2, 470.

The combined New Testament image of Judas hanging from a tree, his bowels out, is an image of a man who's entire being and emotions have exploded outwardly, his existence one of felt ruin and destruction whereby his only felt option was suicide. From Matthew's gospel we read that Judas "changed his heart" (Matt 27:3) and returned the money received from his betrayal of Jesus. And yet events had unfolded beyond his control, and Jesus was going to die. This becomes all too much for Judas, the reality of his actions taking hold of his self, the path of suicide becoming the only way left for Judas to walk, according to his own judgement upon himself.

How significant for us today is Judas' story, then, that there are those of us for whom the only judgement we feel appropriate to render upon ourselves is suicide.

On October 23, 2015, my identical twin brother attempted suicide, an attempt that he thankfully survived. These are his own words as to how he recalls that evening, written ten days after the event,

> "Most days my mind is cloaked in a type of darkness; it is like a black blanket is draped over my brain. It feels as if the underside of the blanket has thousands of tiny hooks which have burrowed into my mind and block feelings of joy, hope, and happiness. The hooks tug and cause an incessant noise which I can't turn off and make me feel as if I am going insane. This 'mind noise' is exhausting and the night I tried to kill myself I felt the only way to silence my mind was to end my life. I felt that to no longer live would be a welcome rest. I felt tired of living. I wanted to die and give my mind peace.
>
> My suicide attempt wasn't planned, it was impulsive, and this scares me. It scares me how easily I went from sitting on my balcony, smoking a cigarette, to walking into my bathroom, finding a large quantity of pills, and taking them. I

did not take the decision lightly, I knew exactly what I was doing, but nevertheless it was an action taken quickly. I know, for many reading this, it is very hard to understand suicide; ultimately, for me, I felt defeated and to carry on living seemed too much. Depression is a continuous, painful battle which is so much more than feelings of sadness or being low. Depression creates a sense of worthlessness, hopelessness, and despair. It is also such an underestimated illness considering the biggest cause of death of men my age (34) in the UK is suicide. Suicide and mental illness are inextricably linked yet the awareness is awfully underwhelming.

It is a blur as to what exactly happened after I took the overdose; there are flashes in my mind of paramedics, being taken to resus at the hospital, drips being inserted, being in and out of consciousness. I have had about ten days to analyze and process what happened that night and I do recall my feelings as I lay on my sofa after taking all those pills. I remember getting sleepy and suddenly panicking that death was the complete and utter end. I remember finding no comfort in the absolute finality of death because I felt I had still achieved so little. I felt so underwhelmed by my life so far, I didn't want to die without having achieved more. I also felt overwhelmed with guilt at the thought of anyone I love discovering me dead; I couldn't do that to them. In a strange sense of irony, I called the emergency services because I felt I had achieved too little in life so far.

As I write this, I am still trying to process what happened; brushing so closely with death does put a lot into perspective though. I am relieved I am still alive because I have a wonderful network of loved ones who are tireless in their care for me. My suicide attempt wasn't me being cowardly or treating life glibly. Rather, it was treating life too seriously and not being able to process it. Suicide is a deeply complex issue, and it wasn't a sudden flick of a switch in my brain. It

> was because of a buildup of circumstance and reflection. It was because of a long battle against darkness and despair. It was because I saw no path forward but only a field of mental thorns. If you are courageously fighting mental illness, then know you are not alone, and I know your pain. Take baby steps each day and I hope and desire you find light amongst the darkness."[1]

The single biggest killer of men in the UK, under the age of forty-five years, is suicide. What's more, eighty-four men kill themselves every week. 75% of all suicides in the UK are men, accounting for nearly 4,500 male deaths by suicide a year. There is something going on within our society that means that twelve men every day take their own life. So, what can Judas teach us to help shed light on, and bring change to, this tragedy?

JUDAS

Judas is portrayed as the ultimate betrayer, the one who sent the Son of God to death. Peter's words in the book of Acts show no sympathy nor grace towards Judas, which is fascinating considering Peter's own denial of Jesus, and the emotional pain and turmoil he suffered when he became aware of his own betrayal of his Lord. It is often said that to understand another's perspective we need to walk in their shoes and share their journey, yet for Peter, Judas is presented as one who got what he deserved for his injustice and betrayal, dying in pain and isolation.

The New Testament speaks of Judas as one whose actions were foretold in Scripture, whose life was "necessary for the scripture to be fulfilled" as Peter says in Acts 1. Yet grasping a

1 https://www.huffingtonpost.co.uk/tom-haward/mental-health-suicide-men_b_8450420.html.

few verses from the Psalms and applying them to the life and events of Judas' life seems a bit of a stretch to then say scripture is being fulfilled! In Matthew's Gospel we are told about the Field of Blood, which was so named because it was bought with the thirty pieces of silver,

> "Then was fulfilled what had been spoken by the prophet Jeremiah when he said, "And I took the thirty silver pieces, the price of the one on whom a price had been set…" (Matt 27:9)

However, this is not a quote from Jeremiah at all; it may be a vague reference to Zechariah 11:3, but the writer of Matthew is being somewhat adventurous with their application. So here in the gospel of Matthew we have the actions of Judas being attributed to a fulfilment of scripture, that is not a fulfilment of scripture at all!

The New Testament speaks of Judas as one whom the devil entered – a thief, traitor, son of perdition, and betrayer. Therefore, we are left with the picture of a man who is utterly appalling, someone of whom we should feel no sympathy, someone who is rotten to the core. Karl Barth says,

> "And no matter how we look at it, we cannot say that the universal expressions of horror with which the New Testament surrounds [Judas] are inappropriate . . . Judas is indeed the "son of perdition," the man into whom the Satan has entered, himself a devil. The New Testament, then, can only reject his repentance, however sincerely he may undertake it."[1]

To read the New Testament, then, is to be left with an image of Judas that is not only a person who should be utterly scorned, but one who should be rejected, one whose

1 Barth, Karl, *CD* II.2, 471.

very life was destined for destruction, whose fate was utter ruin. The figure of a man swinging and spinning from a tree by his neck, swinging with his bowels hanging out, swinging below him in a shorter, quicker arc, is a symbol and picture of what the New Testament and later art leaves us with when we think of Judas. Throughout history, Judas is the very figure of evil and betrayal, one who sent the Son of God to his death. Indeed, in many ways we are left with an utterly "unhuman" picture of Judas, one of whom we should feel little sympathy for. I asked people on social media what images or words came to mind when they heard the name "Judas." Consistently, and unsurprisingly, the answers were, in the main, betrayer or traitor. But what came across even stronger was the sense of tragedy that this name evoked. The people who answered were from a wide variety of backgrounds and beliefs, and yet this name has attached itself within our subconscious leaving us with the overwhelming sense of pain that Judas brings with him. Gone is his life before this act of betrayal, and all we are left with is pain and suffering when we reflect on who he is. Yet he was one of Jesus' closest friends, someone who had walked with him, who had shared meals, laughter, wine, and friendship.

Does not the end of Judas' life reflect one of the great challenges we face with the act of suicide, in that we remember the person because of this final act more than we remember their life before this act? Such is the shock, brutality, and pain suicide brings, it is no wonder that this act can be the lasting impression that we have of someone, an act that seems to almost define them. Yet their life is more than their suicide, and they are more than their mental health. Judas was not simply a man who betrayed Jesus, nor was he simply a man who killed himself: Judas had a story, a life, friendships, joys, victories, failures, hopes, fears, family. Judas was more than the act that ended his life, Judas was more than the tragedy that came to define his life.[1]"

That act of suicide leaves a mark of tragedy upon the person who has killed themselves, upon their own stories, and upon the stories of those who loved them. In the earliest depictions of Christ's crucifixion Judas is seen hanging next to Christ, the death of Jesus bound up in the betrayal and death of Judas. Jesus loved Judas, yet the end of Judas' life is now embedded within our understanding of who Jesus is; the traitor who kills himself and the One of total love betrayed, killed unjustly. Judas and Jesus sit together within our cultural consciousness, tied together in the act of betrayal and death. It is a scene of tragedy.

It is of my belief that this must not be the only picture left, that another story of Judas can be told, a story that can provide insight and hope to men today, men who are dying by suicide every day. Why? Because of those six small words, "Judas had a change of heart . . ."

HOPE

The character Hannibal Lecter delivers a lecture to the Studiolo of the Belle Arti Committee in Florence on the subject of Dante's *Inferno* and Judas Iscariot. In it he makes a link between avarice, treachery, and self-destruction. He says,

1 Karl Barth notes that Judas is described in the New Testament as "one of the twelve," and therefore, his life was as one of the elected, one of those who walked in intimacy with Jesus during his earthly life. He says,

"His election excels and outshines and controls and directs his rejection: not just partly, but wholly: not just relatively, but absolutely. And this is not because it was not really a serious rejection. It is just because it was so serious. It is just because in this figure if in any biblical figure one perceives nothing at all except divine rejection. This very man, who is wholly rejected, is elect." *CD* II.2, 504.

He goes on to say, when summing up about the fate of the rejected (as he puts it), that God's desire is that the Gospel is preached to the rejected and non-elect, that the rejected are not determined by God to remain rejected, but that they are summoned to faith, and that, on the basis of the election of Jesus, they are summoned to believe in their election. c.f *CD* II.2, 506.

> "Avarice and hanging are linked in the ancient and medieval mind: St Jerome writes that Judas' very surname, Iscariot, means 'money' or 'price,' while Father Origen says Iscariot is derived from the Hebrew 'from suffocation' and that his name means 'Judas the Suffocated.'"[1]

Judas, within history, within the arts, within modern parables, is the very figure of self-destruction, not only the betrayer, but one who is a warning to us all of how perilous the road of greed really is. Yet Origen has a different perspective about the man Judas Iscariot, saying that before the soul of Judas was injured by greed and betrayal, it was "quasi a vineyard in blossom."[2] Origen (c. 184 – c. 253) is very sympathetic towards Judas, and sees in his death an act of repentance,

> ". . . the declaration, "I have sinned, in that I have betrayed innocent blood," was a public acknowledgement of his crime. Observe, also, how exceedingly passionate was the sorrow for his sins that proceeded from his repentance, and which would not suffer him any longer to live; and how, after he had cast the money down in the temple, he withdrew, and went away and hanged himself; for he passed sentence upon himself, showing what a power the teaching of Jesus had over this sinner Judas . . ."[3]

Origen brings to light something that occurred in the life of Judas that I believe helps us begin to grapple with the reality of male suicide within the UK, namely, "he passed sentence upon himself. . ." As we heard with my brother's story, shame, regret, and feelings of "worthlessness, hopelessness and despair" becomes the deafening cacophony within the inner lives

1 Harris, *Hannibal*, 935.
2 Comm. on Cant. Cant. IV (lat.) (De- LaRue p. 92)
3 Origen, *Against Celcus*, 2.11, 435.

of those suffering depression and suicidal thoughts; this is the sentence that many are passing upon themselves, one of despair. Having sat for hours upon hours talking on FaceTime with my brother when he was at his lowest, I can tell you that these suicidal thoughts inflict misery upon misery, a debilitating and desperate reality. And yet, paradoxically, the thought of suicide provides a welcome relief. There are those for whom the thought of suicide, the thought of finally being in control in a world of depression where you feel utterly consumed by forces beyond your control, those suicidal thoughts can be a welcome relief, an opportunity to finally feel like there is a way out. In stark contrast to Thomas Aquinas (1225 – 1274) who said that suicide was sinful, a violation to God's order, Nietzsche (1844 – 1900) said, in his work *Beyond Good and Evil*, "The thought of suicide is a strong means of comfort: it helps get us through many an evil night."[1] Nietzsche, in part, saw the voluntary choice to die as a means of establishing our human freedom, and a way of combating the assault of a natural death upon us. Nietzsche did not believe that suicide should be sought out by all, but rather that people should be free to die at the right time. He saw old age death and premature death as both equally unnatural, which is why he said, "Many die too late, and some die too early!"[2] I sympathize with Nietzsche's view, for I have witnessed firsthand the reality of the suffering that many of us are going through, the suffering, pain, and inner tragedy that rages with mental health, and it is no wonder that there are those who desire to find relief. Suicide, though, is not the final word spoken over Judas, and it is not the final word spoken over all have taken their own lives.

Many people feel isolated and alone, and many men are feeling enormous pressure. We have created a society where we have unleashed a monster of loneliness, a sense of

1 Nietzsche, *Beyond Good and Evil*, 157.

2 Z I, On Free Death, KSA 4.93

abandonment, and we are struggling to find ways to provide true companionship, a sense of love and fellowship where we do not feel spurned, where we do not feel as though who we are is a wretch or a failure. Here I am not talking about the need for self-help books, nor '*30 days to the better you*' programs, but a pursuit of what it means to be human, how, in this life, we discover who we really are. Society needs to rediscover, through acts of community, kindness, and genuine friendship, what it means to belong to others, discovering our own somebodiness. Each of us matters, not for what we provide, but for who we simply are.

Judas was not a man who died by suicide; he was, and is, a human with a story, a person of infinite worth.

Bio: Rev Joe Haward is an author, poet, and heretic. As a freelance journalist his work challenges political, societal, and religious corruption, with articles regularly featured in the national news site, *Byline Times*. His fiction and poetry has featured, and is upcoming, in a variety of places, in print and online, including *Outcast Press*, *Cinnabar Moth Publishing*, *No Sell Out Productions*, and *A Thin Slice of Anxiety*. His debut novel, *Burning the Folded Page* (Cinnabar Moth Publishing) will be released in 2023."

WE SHOULD HAVE JUMPED

by Radhika Iyer

I stood by the sofa watching her sleeping. She looked so peaceful, her oily braid hanging over the arm of the chair, her right hand resting on her stomach, and her left hand resting just below her left hip. A pungent mix of coconut oil and talcum powder wafted off her.

I don't know how long I was standing there, watching her. Suddenly her eyes opened, and she gazed at me, devoid of recognition.

I knelt down beside the sofa. "Oh, it's you," she said. "When did you get home?"

"Just a few minutes ago. I didn't want to disturb you because you looked so peaceful sleeping."

She hoisted herself up and looked at the clock. "It's past 2 pm. You should go and have your lunch."

I went into the kitchen and found rice, a lentil curry, and fried cabbage left on the counter. The sink was full of dirty dishes. I heaped the food onto a stainless-steel plate and looked around. I opened a couple of cabinets before I found the rusting milk powder tin tucked behind other tins. I opened it and two *pappadoms* lay at the bottom, still glistening with oil. I reached in and scooped them out, their soft, rubbery texture revealing that they had been lying there for a while. I plonked them onto the mound of food on my plate and came back into the living room, using my right hand to scoop the food into my mouth.

I sat down on one of the single seaters facing her, eating, and looking at her.

"What did you do today?" I asked her, hoping that she would list a bunch of things.

She reached up and undid her braid, letting her hair fall around her face.

"I cooked," she trailed off. "I wanted to do some cleaning but then I felt really tired, so I lay down on the sofa."

I continued to eat.

"Vishnu spoke to me," she said, and looked at me, studying my reaction intently.

"Who is Vishnu? I don't know any Vishnu," I said, speaking with my mouth full, trying to hide the panic in my face and voice, knowing which Vishnu she meant.

"Lord Vishnu," she said, her eyes fixed on me. "God appeared before me and spoke to me."

I wanted to throw the plate of food and scream at her to stop. That God had not appeared to her. That she was hallucinating again.

I swallowed a piece of *poppadom* and felt its edge rub against my throat.

"So, what did Lord Vishnu say to you?" I tried not to sound incredulous.

"He told me not to trust anyone. He said I was right about all the ladies at the association. They don't like me and that's why they are talking about me behind my back and staring at me."

"Which ladies?" I asked, already knowing the answer.

"All of them. All your friends' mothers. They are so stylish, with their hair styles and make up. I don't wear makeup and I don't go to the salon."

"I think some of them are nice to you. I have seen them talking to you pleasantly." I was taking a risk by saying this to her.

"You don't know anything," she snapped suddenly. "You think they are nice, but they are not. If you think they are nice, don't come home. Go and stay with one of them."

"I don't want to stay with anyone else," I said, my eyes filling with tears.

"Then don't say they are nice," she said, but her voice had softened.

I shook my head and wiped my tears away with the back of my left hand.

"Don't cry," she said and reached out to touch my knee. "Keep eating."

"What else did Vishnu say?" I asked.

"I asked him why my life was so bad, and he told me what to do to make things better."

"What kind of things?"

"Some things," she said mysteriously.

I stood up and went to the kitchen. I washed up all the dishes in the sink, tired and angry that I had to come home from school and do housework. I went to the bathroom and saw that the bucket was still brimming with the clothes that I had soaked last night. I always hoped that she would see it and do me a favor just once. I had to hand wash my clothes again. I dared not stuff them into the washing machine anymore. Sometimes clothes remained in that washing machine for a week. That washing machine was more than just a washing machine. I would perch on it some evenings while Mother cooked dinner, chatting with her and asking questions about her childhood in India. Sometimes I would jump off and help her. Once, I had rushed to fry the *pooris*. I had grabbed the doughy circle out of her hand and dropped it into the exposed pan of boiling oil. The oil had splashed on me, hitting my chest, my arms, and my thighs. She had screamed and splashed cold water all over me, asking me again and again if it hurt. I had heard her telling Father later that evening that she hoped I wouldn't have too many scars because who would marry me then?

Father had called a family meeting one evening a few months ago and told us that mother was mad. I was fourteen, my older sister was seventeen, and my younger sister was just six. He told us that she would have monthly appointments with a psychiatrist at the hospital. She would be on medication for a long time.

He looked directly at me and my older sister and said that we would have to do more around the house. Mother would be able to function, but we will have to learn to be independent and take good care of our youngest sister.

He looked at us steadily, waiting for our reaction. We didn't say anything. All I could think was that my mother was mad. She was mad. Would she do stuff like I had seen mad people do on TV? Roll her eyes and laugh hysterically? Tear her hair out in fistfuls? Do even crazier things like run around the house in an unkempt state or worse, naked? Would she come and stand beside my bed while I slept and stare down at me? A shiver ran through me.

Father spoke again, like he had read my thoughts: "Don't let her ill health bother you. You just focus on your studies and activities and do well. Don't let this problem affect your lives." We said okay, of course, for sure. We can do this. Just go on as normal, but maybe do a bit more housework and make sure that baby sister is okay. We could do that.

Father had then leant forward and spoken in a low but stern voice – "Don't tell anyone. Not your friends or anybody. Not anyone at school, not anyone at dance class, no one." We nodded when he paused. "If you tell anyone, you will lose your friends. Because they will say that if your mother is mad, then you will be mad too, one day. Or, no wonder, you are so crazy. They will make jokes about craziness in your family. Everyone will be laughing at you and eventually, they will avoid you." I wondered how my friends would react if they found out about Mother. Would they actually make fun of me? I had some good friends, and they were kind. They wouldn't say such awful things, would they?

But perhaps they were capable of being cruel. When Jaya's brother had killed himself, we had stood in a huddle whispering about it. And then when she had returned to school after a couple of weeks, we hardly spoke to her, avoiding her but staring at her. After a few days, she was back in our clique, quieter than usual but nonetheless, one of us. One Saturday, after badminton club, I was walking towards the school gate when I spotted her behind a tree, looking down at her shoes. "Jaya," I had called out. "You came? But you didn't join us for badminton!" Had she come to school and then hid behind this tree for the whole time?

She had remained silent. I summoned up the courage and said, "Sorry about your brother." She didn't reply. I should have stopped but then I asked, "Did he kill himself?" She looked at me and looked away. She picked up her bag that was lying on the grass and walked away. The following Monday, she was the same as always. That Saturday encounter was never mentioned.

"Can our friends still come round to the house?" I had asked Father. Not that friends came over regularly because of the location of our home – a sprawling area of ten houses, nearly 10 kilometers from the town center, with no public transport. They could only come if their parents agreed to drop off and pick them up.

Father had shaken his head and then changed his mind.

"Yes, they can come but not as often, or they will notice something. Make sure your Mother is in good form before you let them come, and make sure you tell her beforehand so she knows how many are coming, and who is coming so she can prepare. No surprises."

Mother never spoke much to our friends anyway so they would not notice anything amiss. She would usually just say hello when they arrived and later, poke her head into the room to offer snacks and drinks. That's what all mothers did, didn't they? My friends would not notice anything strange.

Where had Mother been the night Father told us about her madness? I could not remember her being in the living room with us. Had she been in bed? In the kitchen? I just could not recall. Maybe she had been doped up with medication and was in bed, sleeping, oblivious of what was going on in the living room.

The next night, after Father had told us the news, he instructed us to switch off the TV and go to our room. It was only 8:30 pm and he very rarely told us to go to bed before 9 pm. We went into our room. We closed the door but opened it again slightly. He was calling somebody. Our phone was located on an old dresser between the living room and dining room. He had pulled up a chair and sat down after dialing the number. By listening, we knew who he was talking to – Aunty Shankar, the most respected woman in our community.

I didn't tell anyone. I spent the next few months being embarrassed of Mother and her behavior. We still attended weddings and other functions hosted by the community. Mother would usually retreat to a corner and sit there for the entire duration. Sometimes other women would go over and speak to her, but the exchange remained brief. My sisters and I would sit with friends, chatting and laughing, and every few minutes, I would look over my shoulder at her. She mostly just sat there, looking down at her lap, her fingers interlaced. Sometimes, I caught her muttering to herself, her head nodding vigorously, her eyes wide and accusing. In those instances, I would quickly turn away, embarrassed, or I would cast a furtive scan around the room, seeing if anybody else was watching her. Sometimes I noticed others staring at her, sniggering, or leaning over and whispering in someone else's ear. I felt ashamed during those functions. Ashamed that I did not have a normal mother, like the other mothers, sitting with their circle of girlfriends, gossiping about scandals in the community, and bitching about other women who were not part of their clique.

But I was also angry. While I gazed at the bride and bridegroom, sweating and repeating chants in front of the *agni* that spluttered and sparked in front of them, trying to look elegant while sitting cross-legged and feeling the numbness spreading along their lower halves, I felt the rage simmer, bubble, and boil within me. I was angry with everyone around us, for seeing the changes in Mother and laughing about it. I was angry with myself for being ashamed of her. I was angry at Father, whom I blamed for her mental deterioration. He had abused her physically and emotionally for years. It was his fault. But most of all, I was angry with Mother. I wanted a mother to care for us and take care of us. I did not want to come home from school, sometimes afraid of entering the house, thinking that I might find her dead on the sofa. Some days, I even hoped that I would find her dead. If she died, the community would rally around us, pitying us as motherless children left behind by a crazed woman, clasp us close to their bosoms, feed us, pamper us, perhaps even adopt us. But of course, I did not want Mother to die. Not because I loved her. Not because she had taught me how to read and write in three languages simultaneously. Not because she had helped me overcome my stutter. Not because she never said I was fat, although

I was fat – the fattest of her children. I did not want her to die because I knew what Father would do.

He would not be able to take care of three girls. He would ship us to India, to live with one of his sisters. Because there were three of us, we might be separated among three households. I thought of his younger sisters in India, my five aunts that I had only met twice. I did not like any of them. They had made snide remarks about how different we were, as we were born and raised in Malaysia. They had imitated our accents and laughed at our pronunciation of certain words. They had criticized our clothes, but then raided our suitcases when we were out and helped themselves to clothes and accessories although Father always presented them with gifts. Their children had called me fat and stupid. I did not want to live in India. I did not want to live with any of them. I sighed with relief every afternoon when I came home from school and found Mother, swathed in a wrinkled, cotton saree, her eyes closed but her chest rising and falling with each breath.

After that evening when Father had told us about Mother, we never spoke of her mental health again as a family. Father would sometimes shout, "You're mad," at her when he was angry with her. He accused her of being lazy and sleeping all the time when he knew that it was the medication that was causing her drowsiness. I went along with this altered norm. My sisters and I did not talk about it either until we were well into adulthood, with jobs, partners, and children. Even then, we only talked about the medication she was on. We did not share our feelings, thoughts, or pain. It was as if we had all decided to obey Father. I cannot speak for my sisters, but I fail to understand why I shut down a whole aspect of my life from the time I was a teenager to adulthood. I told my husband, and later, my children about this experience, but no one else until 2016, when Father passed away.

When I was eighteen, I moved to England to study. During a Friday sleepover with friends, one friend broke down and cried, describing her schizophrenic mother. I could have grasped that opportunity and told her about my mother, too. Instead, I hugged her, uttered suitably consoling words, and reassured her that she could always talk to me. While she was sharing her mum's episodes with me, I was having my own flashback moment to Mother's episodes, telling myself that Mother was not as bad as her mum. Mother could function. She functioned so well that there were times when I forgot she was mentally ill. Or perhaps I chose not to acknowledge it, to pretend she was fine, to block it out. Just because Father said she was mentally ill did not necessarily make her mentally ill. Perhaps, Father had convinced the doctors that she was mentally ill. Seremban was a small town in Malaysia and Father was known by many people. He could have easily fed stories to the doctors. I knew that he had always accompanied Mother when she went into the psychiatrist's office. He never let her go in alone, and he did all the talking. Mother had told me that once when I was home for the summer from England. Mother returned from an appointment at the psychiatric clinic one afternoon. Father dropped her at the door and drove back to work. I was watching TV. She sat on the sofa, adjusting her saree.

"Who is the doctor?" I asked.

"Dr. Shirley George. Her niece was in the same school as you, maybe a year or two older."

I tried to remember someone who I barely knew, and then shrugged my shoulders.

"And what did Dr. George ask you today?"

"She asked me how I was. And I said I was fine."

Mother was gazing directly at the TV while she was talking to me.

"What else?"

"She checked my blood pressure."

"What else did you talk about?"

"Father talked to her."

"What did Father tell her?"

"About what I do every day. About what I did before."

"What did you do before?"

"Some things I did before when I was younger – when we first got married and later, when you were very young."

I waited for more details but there was only silence.

"I am not well in the head," she suddenly announced after a long pause.

I wanted to tell her that she was the way she was because of her life experiences, because of her suffering at the hands of a stranger she had married when she was only nineteen and forced to move to a strange country.

But I did not do any of that. I sat there looking at her, and then said, "I'm sure you didn't do any bad things when you were younger."

"You were very young," she said, her eyes still on the TV.

***

One late evening when the sun was beginning to set, three females were walking abreast towards the Lake Gardens, a huge park at the edge of Seremban town. A woman in her thirties was holding a baby with one arm close to her chest. Her other hand was holding an eleven-year-old girl's hand and that girl was holding an eight-year-old girl's hand. They walked into the park and scooted down a grassy slope until they stood at the edge of the lake.

"We have to jump in," the woman said.

"No," the older girl said.

"I have to die," the woman said, "and I cannot leave you three behind. This is the only way."

"Please Mother! No!" the younger girl screamed.

The baby was quiet.

They stood there for a while, the woman coaxing, and the girls pleading and crying.

Then they walked back home, the dark road lit sparsely by dim orange lights flickering on and off. As they reached the driveway to their house, they saw a man's silhouette standing at the doorway, his hand on his hips. It was too dark to discern his expression.

The baby began to cry, and the woman uttered soothing words.

The two young girls gripped each other's hands tightly, feeling the others' nails dig into their palms.

"We should have jumped," the eight-year-old girl muttered under her breath.

***

I dropped my head into my hands.

"Are you okay?" Mother asked.

I wanted to go over and hold her. Tell her that I remembered. Tell her nothing was her fault. Tell her that I loved her.

But I did not do or say any of those things. I merely nodded, let my hands fall, and without looking at her, I swiveled around to face the TV again.

Bio: Radhika Iyer mainly writes short stories and her first ebook collection of short stories entitled *Why Are You Here?* was recently published by Castles In The Air Press. She has been featured on RTE Radio 1, and her piece, *Am I?* was nominated for Best Short Feature in the 2020 IMRO Radio Awards. Born in Malaysia to migrant Indian parents, she has lived in England and the UAE, and is currently living in Dundalk, Ireland.

MOTHERHOOD IS COMPLICATED

by Kim Jorgensen Gane

I AM FROM ...

I am from Vernon x 4 (one was named Verna); divorced from Phyllis' soprano, who—it was rumored in church choir—harmonized with tenor Grandpa "Tweezer," who planted radishes, prone, one tiny seed at a time.

I am from great freshwater seas whose rip tides swallow swimmers (I once saw the bloated leg of a boy named Brown). Where, on overcast days, you can't distinguish water from sky, good from evil. But poverty from plenty is stark.

I am from Wilfred, "Scotty," of wide smiles and tartan caps, who held us captive for every verse of *Danny Boy*, *Easter Bonnet*, tall tales, and silent flickering 8 millimeters of home; from whose pipe my young fingers poked smoke rings.

I am from loam where English hands grew carrots and grandchildren; upon which I skipped among forsythias beside English heels seeding bluebirds and goldfinches; into which hairless knees over slippered feet pressed pitchforks to reveal new potatoes.

I am from the smell of pickled beets in Lucy's kitchen, the rhythm of her knitting in the orange chair, her irritation with Wilfred's constant pestering, her rings around English rosies, sung in the shallows of Lake Michigan in July.

I am from Pete of silence and church (so he could play softball in summers); from Dorothy of paint and perfection; high school sweethearts I can't seem to embrace at the same time, whose six marriages and five divorces eclipse happier times.

I am from a Mitten surrounded by lakes that fails to keep all its fingers warm or supplied with clean water; a land where disparity blights Black communities, and favors mine, where a lack of public transit fueled by the auto industry keeps us segregated.

I am from my brothers: Vernon the third called "Burt," of the second called Pete. And of David (between my daughters; they were the Musketeers three), born of Dorothy and Ron, who housed my newborn daughter (and me, by default; it was complicated, *he* was complicated).

I am from the stars; from Evergreen to Xanadu, with Midler in between; a songbird without a voice, who played Anna to a King and Mother Nature one Hallows Eve solo, secretly pregnant, broke, broken … now mothering four, a truthteller who won't be silenced.

* * *

I had a recurring nightmare as a child: It started with my brother and me sitting in a parking lot in my mother's Pink Panther pink '69 Mustang convertible. Its white ragtop was down, and its rumble seat was hidden away in the trunk.

The parking lot was outside a crumbling brick building in a southwest Chicago suburb, near where we lived for a couple of years when I was in elementary school. My mom was my Brownie leader. Once, she left us in the car when she ran in to buy patches. I'm sure it wasn't that bad of a neighborhood, but it's also where a cognitively disabled man-child tried to kiss her outside a convenience store. Compared to where we came from, this had a lasting imprint on me.

My brother had once hooked his diapered behind to the gear shifter in my mom's old car. It tumbled down the dirt driveway at my grandparents', with her running after it, shouting at no one, "Stop, Stop!" After my brother dove out the window, she managed to jump in, and the old green Ford Torino lurched to a stop. My mother's white knuckles and heaving breaths are still vivid through the dappled windshield. I suppose I had a well-hidden desire to rescue my little brother from that.

So, my recurring dream took the two of us from that parking lot near Chicago, to a familiar street. Suddenly, we're bouncing along the bluff in our quaint lakeside hometown across Lake Michigan. I am in third grade; my brother is in first. I am behind the wheel of that Pink Panther pink Mustang convertible and we're careening and hanging on for dear life, until I can't keep control on a curve, and we go sailing off the cliff, into oblivion.

Each time I woke, sweating, frightened, and feeling like a failure.

A condition that is oft repeated years later when I'm a single mom, trying to survive with a delightful, sparkly-eyed little toddler to care for. Alone in my conservative hometown. With no child support.

After much convincing, my mother had co-signed a lease for me and my daughter to escape the 1200 square foot house we'd shared with her and her second husband, three dogs, two cats, and my skooching infant half-brother who came a year and nine days after my daughter.

I moved us into a back-alley apartment downtown. It had one bedroom, just wide enough for my daughter's twin-size bed on the floor and an old cane rocking chair from my mother. The room was long and narrow. Her changing-table-turned-dresser occupied one wall, and an overloaded pink metal bookshelf stood just inside the doorway. There was little room for her to play on the floor, and no carpet to cover the distressed hardwood. I read to her in the cane rocker every night before bed, where her projectile spit-up still crusted underneath the swooping wooden arms.

I'd hand-stitched a pink balloon valance for my daughter's room, a blue one for our living room that doubled as my bedroom, and stayed up for almost an entire weekend straight to hand-stitch a blue-flowered comforter for myself. I have it in the guest room to this day. My daughters and their husbands sleep under it when they come to visit from their respective homes in Minnesota and New Mexico. My daughter used to curl up under it on the pullout couch with me. She'd watch Looney-Tunes on Saturday mornings while I slept in.

She'd curl up in my lap on the bathroom floor, and lift my tear-streaked face, and say, "Wudge you, Momma."

It was so hard. Paying for daycare. Keeping the lights on, which I didn't always. Keeping the heat going.

And the loneliness.

A cavernous loneliness from working and earning never enough; from returning bottles and cans from my dad's office for their 5-cent deposit to buy bread and milk and eggs to feed my little girl; from raiding my dad's change jar for quarters to go to the Laundromat to wash our clothes.

There were boyfriends on occasion. We both had our hearts broken more than once before we met the man she would eventually call Daddy. Who walked her down the aisle and cried at her wedding and danced with her under a spotlight into her husband's waiting arms. He gave her an equally impish and delightful stepsister to grow up with, for us to love and to be the only person who could properly send her off to married life with the perfect personalized Maid of Honor song, rapped to the tune of the Fresh Prince of Bel Aire.

Since my husband's daughter, younger by exactly two Januarys, stepped into my daughter's room and said,

"This place is a mess," they've shared every birthday. They've shared Barbies®, Practical Magic, potions, and pets. They've whispered under covers and behind closed doors, over phone lines and across air. They've rescued one another from childhood loneliness, and young adult mishap. They welcomed a long-sought brother into their teenaged lives, whose baby's breath, sweet, meaty little hands, and nighttime cries provided an excellent source of birth control.

Just like their father and me, my daughters are bonded by so much more than blood. They're bonded by history. We're all bonded by exactly what the other needed at precisely the right time.

So, what if…?

What if the recurring nightmare I would remember years later while driving my toddler around that same curve in my 1981 Dodge Omni with no radio; sucking her binky and clutching her soft yellow blankie, her trusting eyes watching me in the rearview…what if instead of putting on the breaks and slowing down and taking that same curve cautiously during a blazing snow-storm and thinking time and again through my tears that long winter that I couldn't possibly do it without her—to leave her with a lifetime of thinking it was her fault? What if I'd closed my eyes, took my hands off the wheel, and decided to just drive into that icy lake?

But I couldn't do it with her either. She was too precious. Too beautiful. Too full of life and possibility and hugs and Wudge You, Mommas. I needed her, and she needed me, and she saved my life in more ways than I can count. But it was all so much more than one girl should have been asked to carry on her tiny shoulders.

We made it through that winter, and another, and another after that. We made it through me losing a job, and my car getting repossessed, and quietly not being able to pay rent the winter after we met her daddy and her sister. We made it to the day we moved into a new place with them, when I saw the weight of more than two thousand days before float off her shoulders with the imagination of two little girls, who were both, for once, just being kids. They were playing with the dollhouse my Gramps had made her on the floor in her new bedroom, which had room enough for two small girls, with the same birthday two years apart, to sprawl out on their bellies.

Thank God I didn't…just drive.

***

I have spent the last year or so on the phone with a dear friend, for up to three, sometimes more hours a day, just trying to keep her alive. To keep her from submitting to society telling her that she doesn't exist, that she should succumb and kill herself. She is a sexual assault survivor. Or, to put it more accurately but less "tastefully," she is a rape survivor.

When I asked her one day whether she thought it was right that I was suicidal when my daughter was young, if it was right that I didn't believe I was worthy of the help I so desperately needed, she said, "No, of course not." And then she sobbed, "But you were a MOOOOMMMM!"

I yelled into the phone, "SO FUCKING WHAT! YOU! ARE A HUMAN! BEING!"

My friend survived lockdown all alone in a house filled with ghosts. The ghosts of her three closest family members who died within a matter of four short years of each other. The ghost of the high school boyfriend who abused her emotionally and sexually when she was only fourteen years old. The ghost of the other high school boyfriend who followed her like a puppy, and who occasionally resurfaces and stalks her still. Literally, there are notes and journals buried under floorboards and behind insulation. She's too afraid to go looking for them. Too afraid of the memories that will surface that she's buried for all these years. I fill in gaps when I can, but we weren't all that close in high school. I try to hold her up and tell the little girl she was that it wasn't her fault. That being too frozen to fight back or to say no plainly—because "STOP" apparently wasn't clear enough—was a completely reasonable response to someone grooming you and telling you that you are worthless all the time.

I was groomed and coerced, too. My own memories aren't always reliable, and my own little girl doesn't always feel equipped enough to go digging.

Except for pure dumb luck, my friend and I are the same: both petite, both gregarious. We both tend to take to a stage and neither of us is afraid of a microphone. We both have tender hearts, a love for and a deep belief in the power of community, and an understanding that we're all in this together—we will sink together, or we will rise together.

Neither of us has a clue which it will be.

* * *

I wrote "Trigger Warning: Mothering Boys" months before the news of the Stanford rapist's sentence infiltrated every social media platform, and rightly so. These were my words, my truth. I wrestled with them. I worked with a writing coach to make better sense of them. To be clear. To find the love in the experience and be able to express that, too.

I read the words before a live audience. My dad was in the audience. My mom was. My brother left before I read my piece. We simply ran too long for his aversion to all things that whiff of "drama" (i.e., girl talk).

My brother is raising four daughters. So, when he cornered me at my niece's birthday party and said, "Dad told me about your talk. I just want the guy's name," I was momentarily taken aback. His posture. His complete lack of compassion, sensitivity, concern. Apology? Maybe?

He said it again, "Tell me the guy's name."

I let out my breath. "I'm not giving you the guy's name, *Fred."

"Why not?"

"Because this is why girls don't tell. Your attitude, attacking me like this. This is why girls don't tell."

"Fine, you're not going to tell me the guy's name? We don't need to talk about it here. I don't do drama."

"Why not? This is the perfect place to talk about it." My hand sweeps the area around the kitchen island, just steps away from where my brother had cornered me, where all four of my nieces were sitting and where all conversation had stopped. "You have four daughters."

My brother says through clenched teeth, "Fine. You want to talk about it. Let's go outside."

I'm shaking. My nails are pressing half-moons into my palms. We sit outside across the fire pit from one another, facing each other like opponents. When aren't we supposed to be on each other's side? Through our parents' divorce and five stepparents we'd managed to pretty much stick together, yet here we were facing one another like this. He was already a little drunk. I had only just arrived.

"Why won't you give me the guy's name?"

"Because this. You. This attitude is exactly why girls don't tell. We don't want someone we love to go to jail. This is completely the wrong response to a situation like this. You're acting like I did something wrong. I'm shaking talking about this with you and it's more than thirty years later."

"Well, it explains a lot, that's all."

I start to think maybe we have a glimmer, "My history. Yeah…"

"No. It explains why you hate men."

I'm stunned.

"That's not fair," I sputter. "I do not hate men. I love men."

"Well, everything you post [on Facebook] makes it pretty clear you hate men, and now I know why."

"I do not hate men. I love men. I'm actually married to a pretty evolved guy, a feminist even. I'm raising two boys. I do *not* hate men." I'd worked so hard to find the love in my story. The love for my two then 13-year-old boys who had triggered fears in me of screwing up and raising boys who would commit sexual assault, or any kind of assault, violence being something my dad and brother still access easily.

I'd stuck with my husband through two cross-country moves, two downsizes, closing a restaurant and bankruptcy, his depression and, I suspect, being suicidal. I'd even worked to find compassion for my rapist, for whom clearly no one had ever defined rape or sexual coercion. He was the son of a single mom. They were poor. He had no male role model. These weren't conversations we were having in 1983.

I had hoped to make a difference in that conversation today, in this age of promposals and sexting, for my boys and the girls they will encounter. Yet my dad hadn't **received** that deeply important message from my "talk," and he certainly hadn't relayed it to my brother. And my brother hadn't even bothered to ask to read it.

It was a deeply troubling conversation with someone I love.

And then news of the Stanford rapist came out. And I felt validated. Yet, even more troubled at what an incredibly long uphill road we must conquer.

I look behind me, over the last thirty-plus years, and I'm not even sure we're at the mid-point. But I know with even more certainty how important my contribution is to the conversation. And I get another wind.

* * *

I know from experience that the moment we stand upon the precipice of motherhood, looking down one perilous side and then the other, neither presenting a particularly soft landing, we are mothers. The call to mother is consuming, as is the fear and the shame and the desperation of not wanting to mother. Or not wanting to mother again. Not wanting to fail yet another helpless soul. Between exists everything from ambivalence to joy, from denial to eventual acceptance. All children are blessings, yes, of course. But all pregnancies are not. And only a pregnant person can know which is true with each pregnancy, each circumstance.

What I didn't express to my brother was how angry I was and remain. How angry I've always been. I didn't get to say, having been a single mom working two low-wage jobs myself, how viscerally I understand poverty and that it keeps women from participating in our economy and in our government. I didn't get to talk about the second time I was sexually assaulted, in student housing near Western Michigan University's campus.

Or, as they near a close, how deeply I've experienced the entirety of my childbearing years avoiding pregnancy, my abortion, raising children, and for six years before my son was born when my girls were teenagers, trying desperately to *get* pregnant, including surviving a miscarriage, and believing at the time that it was the penance I had to pay for a sexual history I didn't always choose.

What I couldn't embrace myself, because I hadn't found it yet, was my truth: that I am a survivor.

Women hold treasures far more valuable than brute strength: flexibility, common sense, diplomacy, the ability to multi-task and keep entire families together, to balance and stay within budgets, to go Momma Bear, Tiger Mom, and even Hockey Mom and fight to the death for our clan when we must. We do this while our men-folk bump chests, bully, and bluster, and attempt to bend the world with their military prowess, to bend us with their physical strength. Women are cut open or ripped open to give birth; we survive rape, breast cancer, poverty, and oppression.

We possess strength beyond their imagination, and it terrifies them.

***

I believe I was raised to feel powerless. As a single mom for the first six years of my daughter's life, as a sexual assault survivor, I felt like a victim. I internalized religious shame. Having been born "female," I deeply felt being oppressed. I shared this information when I was in a Brave Talks training facilitated by Demetrius of the YWCA in Kalamazoo—Kalamazoo, where so many of my secrets were buried until I started sharing my story—who said, "We cannot hope to achieve gender equity without also healing racism." His words changed everything for me. Working on these issues in concert—being in the work together, in healthy ways, especially with women of color—has become my North Star.

Bio: Kim Jorgensen Gane is a speaker, writer, storyteller, and activist from Michigan. She is writing her book, *Mother Activist: Raising Ourselves and the Men We Fall For, A Love Story*, because the brother she loves so much is an alcoholic who's never had permission to define himself either. She is a two-time PechaKucha St. Joseph/Benton Harbor presenter.

SEE ME

by Mike Hickman

Five, nearly six, months away from work and the fear of being seen had still not diminished. If anything, it had only gotten worse. Once, I'd had a choice in how much was seen. Now, my best option was the perpendicular.

There was a time when I was adept enough to hide the majority of my socially awkward tics. So, even though walking down the road and spying anyone I knew in a professional or non-professional context caused me to die a million agonies inside, I could – at a push – summon up enough energy to paste the expected smile on my face. I could just about manage to shuffle my much-abused set of Socially Acceptable Response cards, maybe mustering a half convincing "hello" or even brazening out the whole, "I didn't see you there because I was so totally engrossed in my MP3 player, my reflection, my shoes, the sudden appearance of that lamppost in my path."

Douglas Adams and John Lloyd's *Meaning of Liff* has a word for that moment of decision as you determine whether to acknowledge someone approaching (is it "Droitwich"?[1]) and it certainly deserves one. It was always an anxiety minefield for me, even before the worst happened, and it was so easy to get wrong. On days when "hello" was too much, I might, for example, entirely

---

1 Oh, by the way, I was wrong about Droitwich, too. The moment when two people recognize each other and pretend they haven't is a "corriearklet". There, you feel better knowing that, don't you?

overdo the studied blanking thing. Maybe I'd stop and stare at passing squirrels or take a very particular interest in that *Buy One Get One Free* offer in the shop I had not noticed and wouldn't have shopped in even if I'd had the money. And I knew this would not go unremarked. If anything, I was outright inciting the "I saw you this morning…" speech in front of my colleagues. The logic was always very straightforward – they had seen me, so there could be no reasonable excuse for me not seeing them in return. And I'd think of all the excuses, and I'd know that it was perfectly reasonable to have missed them waving at me – most especially as they'd no right to my attention anyway; no employment contract can demand that much. I could claim to have legitimately missed them, but then I would feel shamed because there was no way to make that lie retrospectively true. I had determined that I couldn't deal even with so much as a "hello," and all while knowing that they had invested their energy in noticing me, perhaps preparing their own "nice day" or "funny seeing you here" or any number of other greetings that, truth be told, as much irritated me with their lack of sincerity and meaning as I irritated myself with my permanently switched on sense of shaming self-consciousness.

So, yes, I could definitely do the studied blanking thing. I could definitely reach for that option if it was – dear Lord – Deborah, who always noticed *too much*, or Suzanne or Andy or James, who noticed nothing like enough but didn't let it stop them presuming who I was and where I was going and what that ought to mean. I could tough them all out. But then, almost immediately, and well in time for what I would have to suffer when I next saw them, the resentment would start. Yes, you *did* see me there. Ha, ha, ruddy ha. Yes, I somehow failed to notice you, even as you gave me the full-on semaphore greeting from across the street, so I must have had a lot on my mind, mustn't I? I must have had my head in the clouds, mustn't I? How unutterably inexcusable of me. And how impossible for me to say what was really in my mind or why bumping into someone I knew was as welcome as a surprise trepanation with a blunt wood chisel.

Why didn't you see me? That's what they'd be asking. They'd fulfilled their end of the deal. So why hadn't I?

Because I *did not* want to be seen.

Because I knew they wouldn't see me, anyway.

Because, even if I had acknowledged them, I'd still have wound up with some variation of this: "I saw him on his way to the shops/out for a walk/in his civvies."

"I can prove he exists outside of the workplace."

"I saw who he is, really."

Except they hadn't. That's why I wouldn't want to be truly seen by them, because then they would know more than just where I was going (as if that could ever be important), what I was up to (very much ditto), and why I'd left the house dressed quite like that or bought those particular items from the supermarket (wasn't I supposed to be on a diet? What was with all the crisps?)

Maybe I'm telling you too much. Maybe this is all just me. Very likely. But the fact remains that, even before What Happened ™, this was often the best I could manage. The self-conscious "hello" or the thorough blanking before being outed, even shamed, the next day for it.

There was an assumption on their part, I thought, that they had to be the problem. That I wasn't noticing them because of something they had done.

It was as if there couldn't be anything else on my mind at all that might have blocked them out. Or blocked out the thoughts of me in work, as that person, in that shirt and tie, with that smile and that voice and those stories that were all designed – wasn't it just the same for them? – to cover the me that I couldn't take in with me, that I had to keep hidden, that I knew would repulse them as soon as they saw him.

It was so often easier just to say "hello."

That is, until What Happened™, happened. It was over a year before I ventured outside again after the sojourn in the Cedar Ward and, then, only for my prescribed group therapy sessions, 9:30 am on a Monday and 2:00 pm on a Thursday (scheduled as if to cause maximum disruption to the members – if you were working, good luck trying to get those slots off twice a week; if you weren't, good luck trying to arrange the rest of your life around them).

The venue for group therapy was – of course it was – in a run-down terraced house, leased I suppose by the NHS, in the middle of town. Right in the middle. "Slap bang," as they say, giving few options in terms of the approach that had to be made at such prime times in the day. Giving rise to maximum risk of Adams' and Lloyd's Droitwich somewhere *en route*.

I could no longer manage even the mumbled "hello" option, standing there, shuffling, as my would-be interlocutor's pupils attempted to fix my own in place – *you will* not *look away while I'm talking to you, although, if you do, I'll just stand here and quiz you some more*. I had to come up with an alternative.

Which is where perpendicular came in.

In the past, I'm sure I might perhaps have unconsciously sought the perpendicular option. Ducking down the side road that added another ten or fifteen minutes to my journey, but was far less travelled by anyone I happened to know. So, there'd be no agonies over recognizing or not recognizing people. No agonies about whether to take my glasses off or dash them to the ground as excuse-ahead-of-time for not seeing them. No anxiety over recognizing or not recognizing people or what to do with my face at a distance, and whether I could maintain the same expression until they were upon me.

Perpendicular offered me an instant win, and such a win that I hadn't realized its power.

And this sort of thing was, on occasion, going on when I was "well." When I was lecturing sometimes up to 150 students at a time (a nightmare vision in itself for some, I know). When I was presenting at conferences in countries whose languages I couldn't speak and chairing meetings and performing in amateur theatre. Quite a lot of the people I was interacting with would have been surprised at my automatic perpendicular propensities when I was so visibly dealing with all of that.

But, after I received my "working diagnosis" from the friendly neighborhood psychiatrist and I was signed off sick, I found myself more than ever before conscious about the whole business of being seen. Not just on the street as my sort of perhaps real self, if we presume that I ever let him out of the house, but out *at all*. And this was not just because this might mark me down as a malingerer – although, of course, anything more than nipping to the post box and the informers would have tipped off HR – but because now – *now* – it wasn't just me that didn't want to be seen. I'd had confirmed what I had always suspected – my colleagues did not want to see me.

That delight they once took in asking where I was going, what I was doing, how it was possible to buy a packet of crisps quite that big, was now replaced with a palpable sense of discomfort that I was still out there at all. Now they were the ones dropping their gaze, examining their toecaps, taking time to explore the hedgerows, getting up close and personal with the streetlamps. Anything, *anything*, to avoid acknowledging that we existed in the same world, let alone the same on the same pavement.

And I remembered my predecessor in that job succumbing to mental health issues (coincidence? Hmmm…) and how people talked about her being seen about when she was off work. Someone had spied her in a well-known, and rather swanky, tea-room. It was reported back to other colleagues in words that dripped with suspicion and insinuation. It was, I thought then, as if she wasn't allowed any kind of existence beyond the ill health house arrest. I thought it was unnecessarily snarky and who were they to police what she did when she was working towards a recovery that ultimately turned out to require her resignation and relocation to the other end of the country.

But what I missed – what I didn't know until it happened to me – was their anger. They didn't want to be reporting that they'd seen her in *Bettys* with someone who looked suspiciously like she might have been a friend. (A friend! Imagine it! Allowed a friend when recovering from a mental health crisis. How very dare she! The prospect that it might have been a Community Psychiatric Nurse or similar hadn't occurred to them. But, then, they'd not yet encountered that world, knew nothing of what they might discover there – *and they had no intention of ever doing so*). They did not want to be forced to think about what it must be like. They wanted her to be elsewhere. In that ward they'd heard of, perhaps, where there were locked doors and – hadn't someone told them? – bars on the windows. They wanted her to be out of sight because she was out of her mind. And there was no way they wanted to trouble theirs with what she might be up to.

"You don't know that's what they're thinking," Group Therapy Christopher argued, when I attempted to describe the look of something not altogether related to disgust that now crossed my soon-to-be former colleagues' faces when they realized that I might be heading their way.

"They could be thinking about any number of things. The washing. Their day. It doesn't have to be about you."

And I'd have believed that, perhaps, if it hadn't been for the way they'd been over Helen. I'd have thought it was my paranoia or over-sensitivity talking when I obsessed about the whispers behind my back. But they weren't just whispers behind my back. It was there on their faces. Right from the very first people I encountered in the silent weeks after coming out of the ward and needing to make my way outside again. Both times, the colleagues in question risked a full-on look at me before very, very pointedly and very, very obviously deciding that it was for the best if I was not seen. One hesitated a fair bit before making this decision – I could see how torn he was between pretending I wasn't there and just coming over and saying something. But both ultimately ended up making the same call. Both carried on their business of walking past me with a very concentrated air of being Really Very Interested In Anything But Me.

And, somewhere, I could understand this. If someone has been away from the workplace for a while and they're no kind of friend, whatever their role in relation to you, it's going to be very, very difficult to strike up any kind of conversation. The words "how are you?" were hardly used within the institution I worked for. The Head Honcho in my faculty found it difficult to say those three words even when he could have been reasonably assured that the person he was asking them of was in good shape and feeling fine. Now imagine how hard it is to say anything at all when the person you're speaking to is off ill with what has been formally identified on sick notes as "anxiety" but actually goes rather further than that. Not easy. There are so many, many ways to put your foot in it. So many, many ways to add to the awkwardness. So, it was altogether better just to take a deep breath and file the sick colleague into the mental folder marked "Somebody Else's Problem." All perfectly understandable. All perfectly painful. All perfectly avoided by taking that perpendicular turning.

The trouble was, back in the days when my life still had wheels, not being seen, as I've illustrated, was something I actively sought out. If they could join me in my fiction that we were, the pair of us, independently making our way to work in our own bubbles and there was no necessity to acknowledge anyone else's existence at all, then I'd tell myself I was happy (I told myself I was happy over any number of things – this may or may not have been part of the problem). Now, the realization that they *did not want to see me* was painful. I wonder if it's the equivalent of Eddie Izzard's lovely "no information on this" routine (the shopkeeper faced with Eddie being Eddie at the head of his queue has a sudden mental fugue and is incapable of doing anything but moving the *Twixes* round the back…). If the troubled-by-my-presence-outside-in-the-real-world colleague had any knowledge that the sick notes said "anxiety," they didn't know how they were supposed to respond when the person labelled that way was suddenly *there*, large as life, on the pavement in front of them. If they didn't know why I'd been away for such a long time, it was even more problematic. What could they say? Anything could potentially turn into the verbal equivalent of a landmine. It was best not to say anything at all.

And then there was my feeling that the mental weather of depression and anxiety is just not seen properly, if at all. To have that proved, in public, and to be the one that is so very pointedly not seen, is discomforting to say the least.

I'd sometimes wonder whose mind I was trying to ease, taking the perpendicular path. I know how hard it was to see them blank me. I know how hard it was to have a point proved about my former behavior towards them. Behavior that I couldn't, then, have interrogated any further. I know that it benefited me. But I did not want to be seen, remember? Wasn't that where we came in? I was supposedly okay with it.

And then it hit home, as it had to – I was doing it for them. I was trying to be sensitive to their fear of being seen. To their fear that what had happened to me – and what might, therefore, so easily happen to them – might be seen in their faces.

Five, nearly six, months away from work and the fear of being seen had still not diminished. If anything, it had only gotten worse. But my own fear, as a result of that thought process, was well on the way to diminishing. With help from the perpendicular path.

Bio: Mike Hickman (@MikeHicWriter) is from York, England. He has written for Off the Rock Productions (stage and audio), including a 2018 play about Groucho Marx and Erin Fleming. Since 2020 he has been published in *Agapanthus* (Best of the Net nominated), *EllipsisZine*, the *Bitchin' Kitsch*, the *Cabinet of Heed*, *Sledgehammer*, and *Red Fez*.

FUNCTIONAL

by Kiersten Lipps

I once took part in a study on specialized treatment for cross-sectionality of symptoms of depression and OCD.

"You?" a co-worker asked when I tried to explain the study. "I didn't know there was anything wrong with you."

Most people don't. All my illnesses are invisible.

You can't see when my heart begins to race from anxiety, or when my mind hyper-fixates on a meaningless, passing conversation thanks to OCD, or when I feel like I can't breathe because I'm questioning my self-worth due to depression, or when my fibromyalgia sends roving pain through my body.

Functional.

That's what it's called when you've learned to continue a conversation through the panic attack, to disguise the compulsion as organization and cleanliness, to smile through the depressive thoughts, and to work through the pain.

People mistake it for mildness, that my symptoms—my illness—must be lesser. One time I scored myself high on an anxiety test and the doctor made me retake it with assistance. This time they talked through each question with me, explaining it in detail and then rating each scaled score based on my answer. Turns out, I'd graded myself too low the first time. Granted, I was irate the second time I took the test given that the doctor hadn't believed me, hadn't trusted my own analysis of my anxiety. Who was he to judge what was happening in my mind? All he had to judge me on was the still surface, he couldn't see the current of anxious thoughts and habits flowing underneath.

That study I took part in, it required intensive interviewing to establish a personalized questionnaire about my symptoms—they not only accepted my test results but took a closer look. The questions were based on my specific symptoms, which meant they ranged from 'Did you use a public bathroom today' and 'I controlled my fluid intake to avoid using a public bathroom' to 'I had feelings of self-doubt' and 'I felt anxious about how others viewed me.'

I had to complete the personalized questionnaire three times a day for nearly a month. The results were then turned into an associative map—basically the idea was to determine which intrusive thought or compulsion started the domino effect of the others. Then, they could target the primary behavior in an attempt to reduce the other symptoms as well. I was convinced they would cure my phobia of public bathrooms – It's not the germs; I think I'm going to be killed in a stall one day.

"We spent hours looking at your map," the doctor told me. "Another participant gave us permission to show you theirs so you can see what a normal one looks like."

Even my mental illness is abnormal.

Apparently, most people develop two distinctly separate symptom clouds. The OCD symptoms working independently from the depressive symptoms.

Not mine. Mine was an enormous jumbled mess, all the symptoms overlapping and echoing off each other. I obsess about intrusive thoughts born of my depression and anxiety. The more I fixate, the more the anxiety and depression symptoms increase and so on and so on.

They couldn't explain the bathroom thing. It was all alone—its own separate, inexplicable fear. So I continue to monitor my fluid intake so that I can continue to go 8-10 hours between bathroom breaks. I only use single stall restrooms or my home bathroom. My record for holding it to avoid using a public restroom is 16 hours—a road trip after work. One friend insists my bladder is just going to give out one day, another encourages my bravery on the rare occasion I simply must use a public stall by calling out, "Don't get got." Whatever the cause of the fear, it was unresolved by the study.

The benefit of my unusual map, however, was that they could target my depression, anxiety, and OCD symptoms all at one time by targeting a single behavior.

All in all, it was pretty effective.

I learned how to recognize an intrusive thought, how to challenge it, wrangle it back so my day wasn't completely sidetracked by what a healthy mind would dismiss out of hand. They taught me to retrain my thinking habits. That is, instead of having an intrusive thought and then ruminating on it all day, I can now recognize when I'm having an intrusive thought and then analyze it: What triggered this thought? Is this thought logical? Do I have evidence to suggest this thought is true? Usually no, usually it's just my mind jumping to the worst possible conclusion. But, on the rare occasion my thought is based on evidence, I then ask—what steps can I take? What's within my control?

A healthy mind does this a bit more naturally—intrusive thoughts happen to everyone, after all. The key difference is that with OCD and Generalized Anxiety Disorder, the thought is sticky (i.e., instead of just dismissing or ignoring the thought, my mind lingers on it). With the help of my doctor in the study, I learned to capture these thoughts and release them—with moderate success. It takes practice to learn to moderate your own thinking. I've gotten pretty good at it in the years since the study.

Still though…

It's over a hundred degrees outside, in the middle of September, and I have just finished wrapping nine Christmas presents. I send a picture to friends and family, as I'm particularly proud of the wrapping job.

"You make me sick; it's not even October."

"Wow! You're so organized and on top of things!"

"You're living three months ahead."

That last one slams into me. Compliment though it was meant to be, I am struck with the realization that I have allowed an obsessive behavior of mine to get out of hand. I plan and plan and plan my life to an unhealthy degree.

People mistake this for organization, attention to detail, even as ambition or dedication. In reality, it is an unchecked symptom of anxiety and OCD. An attempt to control the unknown and the future, because if I can control the situation, maybe I can control my symptoms.

I hyper-fixate on Christmas every year—overwhelmed by a desire to give a gift that will be validated as 'good' and therefore validate *me* as 'good'. Honestly, I should start giving out gift cards—everyone loves them and it'd be a lot less to think about. Instead, I start planning and Christmas shopping every July, and let it build and build and build until my husband has to gently tell me it's enough. *I'm* enough.

That was the big takeaway from the study. My number one intrusive thought is a doubt of my self-worth. The first attempt at treating this symptom was to convince me that I have worth inherently due to my being a living, breathing person. "Life," they said, "has inherent value. Human life especially so." I argued for nearly an hour with the lead doctor in the study that human life is not inherently valuable, that we must *do* something with the gift of life to be *worth* something.

When I repeated this argument to my regular therapist, she asked, "Why do we need to be worth something at all? Can't you just live and die and have fun in between and that be it?"

This is why I love my therapist. She doesn't waste my time arguing with me about definitions; she just shifts the perspective a bit. I still don't have an answer to her question—but it was a paradigm shift for me. The idea that I could just live without proving myself to anyone or leaving anything behind when I die, and that'd be okay, that was a freeing thought. I don't owe the universe anything for my existence—it's okay to just focus on my own quality of life. This is something I must remind myself of frequently.

I wonder sometimes if healthy minds spend days and weeks fixated on such thoughts, or do they accept their place in the universe with a shrug and move on? Lost in such thoughts, my more physical OCD symptoms will go unchecked—I run my tongue methodically over the backs of my teeth, pick at the scabs on my scalp from where I picked it open last time, absently count my steps or ceiling tiles, line up the items in front of me—even if they don't belong to me.

Perhaps my symptoms *are* less intrusive to my life than others. Smaller and more discrete, pocket-sized mental illness for a girl on the go.

But it's still there. Functional, invisible, mild as it may be—it's still there preventing me from achieving my best, still present every moment of my life, a factor in every decision I make. I can do everything right: take my meds, eat well, exercise, get lots of rest, socialize, use my coping skills—but I'm still ill. Even if others can't see it, I'll still be battling myself every day.

When I was in graduate school, I asked the nurse practitioner in my primary care doctor's office for a temporary handicapped placard. "I don't need it every day," I explained, "but some days I just can't make the walk across campus. My legs just hurt too much sometimes, and I never know when the next flare is going to happen."

She declined my request.

I seemed healthy enough to her, was able to walk into the office just fine, even walked for exercise—clearly I was just trying to avoid paying for campus parking. My physical illness, like my mental illness, isn't obvious to the seeing eye and exists on its own schedule. It can be easy for people to forget I have these mental and physical illnesses. Even my own husband is sometimes surprised when I suddenly reach a breaking point.

Once, when we were travelling overseas, I had exhausted my tolerance for new experiences. I needed something familiar, so we stepped into a McDonalds. I took one look at the menu in those foreign characters and completely broke down, overtaken by panic and exhaustion. My husband could not fathom why I was crying and hyperventilating over the process of ordering chicken nuggets.

His shock stems from my ability to mask my symptoms. I'm very talented at hiding my duress until I simply cannot take another step, complete another task, or fake another smile. These breakdowns—often appearing as sobs and tears, sometimes as a raging temper tantrum—seemingly come out of nowhere and are triggered by seemingly innocuous things. I once threw an entire meatloaf across the kitchen and damaged the pan, all while screaming like some feral animal. For the life of me I can't remember why I was so angry in that precise moment, likely a misplaced item or some other minor inconvenience.

What matters is what led up to the moment, the hours, days, or even weeks beforehand of anxiety, doubt, obsession, depression, and physical pain brought on by my illnesses.

It is easy for even the people who know me well to forget there is something wrong beneath the surface. Some days I hurt worse, am more anxious, or bluer. But the symptoms are always there to some degree. I'm never not in pain. Never not anxious about something. Never not hyper-fixating on something. The degree just changes. So too does people's tolerance for my differences.

Before I started my medication I was more impulsive in making brash, negative statements and voicing my general opinion. I can recall the relief from my mother-in-law when I told her I was about to start medication—maybe then I wouldn't "ruin"so many family events. She never understood why I couldn't just ignore the casual racist, bigoted, or womanizing comments from other family members.

"Why do you always have to pick a fight?"

"Don't worry," I assured her. "I'll be a little less myself soon. I'm starting a new medication."

"Well that will be good for everyone," she answered with a laugh.

And isn't that a painful joke? My therapist had spent so much time convincing me that my own mind was tricking me into thinking others disliked me, but here was confirmation of my fears. The raw, true me? That person isn't pleasant—even I can't stand her.

Neither can my bosses.

I've been told my mind works at a much faster pace than others. Not in the sense that I can solve math equations fast or play chess well—I can do neither of those things—but that when I am asked to implement something, I often "predict" potential problems very quickly.

My bosses think I am just being negative, nit-picky, or a nay-sayer when I raise my hand in staff meetings announcing new procedures or policies and ask, "But what about when…" I don't mean to be a pessimist, I'm not trying to make my administrators look foolish or unprepared. I genuinely want to know what to do.

What's happening is that while the healthy minds in the room are learning about the new policy or procedure, considering its benefits and how the changes might affect them, my mind is running scenarios through my head, imagining the implementation process. It's part of that echo chamber of anxiety and OCD to be constantly asking, "But what if…"

'What if a student does X, how does that affect the policy?'

'The policy says to do Y, but what if I don't have the tools to do that?'

'The new policy suggests Z, but that contradicts this other random law I happen to remember from when I was fixated on knowing student legal rights.'

Apparently, my bosses don't appreciate this kind of feedback in front of an audience. I've been written up, lectured, and once, it was highly recommended to me that I quit my job if I couldn't be more positive. All of these events were triggering to me, causing panic attacks of one nature or another. It was difficult for me to understand. For years I struggled with processing why I was in trouble for asking a simple question. I wasn't being negative, I genuinely wanted guidance or understanding.

"So tell them that," said my therapist, "and start writing your questions down instead of blurting them out."

Learning to bite my tongue was difficult, but I learned not to compulsively ask my questions—the answers could wait. Then, after the meeting with the team or faculty, I would approach with my list of questions. A principal who had once written me up for "unprofessional behavior" for speaking out of turn in meetings actually became accustomed to me approaching him with my list. Then, one day he came by my classroom before rolling out a new policy. He wanted to hear my questions ahead of time—"They really help me improve our plan." That interaction empowered me, my illness and unusual thought process was actually a benefit and asset.

Other bosses in the future didn't see it that way, though.

My last year working in a brick-and-mortar school building—I work virtually now—my principal was pushing "positive mindset." The atmosphere he created was one of toxic positivity, one in which negative emotions were simply not valid or tolerated. My questions were seen as defiance, my depressive and anxious symptoms as dramatics, and my burnout of the profession as an attitude problem. Everything, in this man's eyes, could be fixed by simply looking at things in a more positive way—which meant no problems ever got fixed at all.

At the advisement of my therapist, I wrote an email. I discussed that his version of positivity was, in fact, toxic, and that for those among the faculty like myself it was a slap in the face to our mental illness. I cannot cure my anxiety through good thoughts, I cannot rid myself of OCD by looking for a silver lining, and I cannot banish my depression with a good attitude. My brain, even with medication, simply doesn't work that way. Sometimes people are sad, or angry, or frustrated and those emotions need to be validated instead of ignored. To demand positivity 100% of the time is discrimination.

That principal didn't speak to me directly for the last few months of the school year. A week after I sent the email, the head principal called me into her office to suggest I quit my job and seek employment elsewhere.

"You're obviously not happy enough here," she said. "So you should go."

They didn't understand, or perhaps they didn't believe me. After all, I don't look sick. I don't fit the stereotypes of the mentally ill. My struggle is a relatively quiet and personal one.

Mental illness takes many forms. It is not something easily defined or diagnosed, and each and every case is unique to the mind it belongs to. Regardless of how it manifests, at what severity, the experiences of the mentally ill are valid and worthy of recognition. We are not lesser for our differences.

Bio: Kiersten Lipps lives in West Texas where she has been a high school English teacher for over a decade. She holds a B.A. in English with a focus on teaching and a Master's in Public Administration. In her role as a teacher, Kiersten has placed an emphasis on the mental health and well-being of her students—helping her campuses to kick-start Social Emotional Learning curriculum and providing students with a safe space to be themselves no matter their differences.

HOLLOW LEG

by Em Frappier

I turned 40 this year – a birthday that is dreaded by many. Women especially. We're supposed to believe that our decline begins at 40, that we will become more and more insignificant as the years accumulate past this arbitrary point. Personally, I never believed I would reach this age. I made no plans for this part of my life because I was convinced I wouldn't make it.

I almost didn't.

I've battled with my mental health for my entire life. Even as early as five years old I knew something was wrong with me. I knew I was broken. Growing up I was not allowed therapy or medication. Not even after I swallowed a bunch of pills in an effort to end my horribly painful life. My cry for help fell on deaf ears, and I was labeled emotional, crazy, and a disappointment. Imagine waking up from a failed suicide attempt to hear how disappointed your father was with you.

Disappointed in what? That I tried? Or that I failed?

I'll never have an answer to that question. My father passed away three and a half years ago from a rare type of cancer. This is when I truly hit rock bottom. I was never that far away from the bottom, though I didn't understand that at the time.

As the end approached, I was shoved back into the old family dynamic and spent ten days watching my father die, trying to comfort him, and taking the brunt of my family's pain. That was my job. If I am a worthless, messed up person, then they are fine. Better than me, anyway.

It was hard to take it all in and grieve while also being admonished for crying. Feeling unwanted by everyone else surrounding my father's bed was not unusual, but I had hoped I might be spared that treatment during a time of such duress. I wanted so badly to help them all feel better. I wanted to take their pain away. I thought I could back then. I thought it was my responsibility. Every single moment of those ten days was torture. At the time, I thought it was just grief. I still refused to see the truth of my situation.

When he did eventually pass, I returned to my own family and my roles of wife and mother, but things were so heavy and so dark. I spent a year barely able to get out of bed and crying sporadically throughout the day. For an entire year I barely existed, yet I rallied every weekend when my mother would visit. I would listen to her rant for hours. We never spoke about my father. She never once asked me how I was doing. It was as if I had not lost my father. As if I had not sat at his bedside for days. As if I couldn't possibly be grieving.

After a year in the darkness, I knew I needed to make a choice. Death or finding a way to fix my brain. Now, my kids are my life, and I could never put them through that kind of pain. Finding help had to be my choice. I was scared. I was raised to believe that therapy was only for the very worst of people – the hopeless cases – but now I was one. Therapy seemed to be my only hope.

My first attempt was terrible. I met with a woman who had lost her dad as well. In fact, he had passed after my father. Her pain was newer than mine. She loved her dad very much, and she immediately assumed that my relationship with mine was the same. She kept making assumptions and telling me stories about her dad. She cried.

I wanted to discuss my binge eating and history of eating disorders. It was during one of the peaks in my disorder. My life was an endless cycle of bingeing to numb the emotional pain until I was in immense physical pain. I spent the next day feeling sick with a food hangover, which led to guilt, which led to another round of bingeing. And repeat. Forever.

When I tried to talk about it, she blew it off. She said that everyone eats a whole bag of chips at one time or another. Yes. That's true. But does everyone eat everything in sight, without tasting or feeling anything, until they are in physical pain and on the verge of vomiting? No. No, they don't.

I tried to ghost her after one session. She sent me emails for a month, even after I told her that I would not be seeing her again. She was rather aggressive and put me off therapy for another six months.

Meanwhile, I kept getting sicker. The world kept getting darker.

My husband was worried, but he had no idea how to help me. I didn't have an answer for him. I believed I was born broken and unfixable. Still, he convinced me to try again. I went back online and got another referral.

This one was a woman I vaguely knew. I live in a very rural area. Everyone knows everyone, and I had met her a few times before. It was years ago. I didn't know if she would even remember me. I tended to believe that people forgot me as soon as I walked away. There was even a period in college when I seriously wondered if I was invisible. I felt like a ghost.

I was nervous about seeing someone I knew, even minimally, but something told me to give it a try. She was away and couldn't see anyone for two weeks, but I made an appointment anyway. At least I had some idea of who she was, unlike the last one.

Listening to my gut at that moment was the best thing I have ever done for myself. She is the perfect therapist for me, and with her patient guidance, I have finally found a little peace. I have realized that while I may have been broken, it was not entirely my fault, and with consistent effort I could heal.

I have always been fascinated by psychology, and this led me to dive deeper and try to learn everything I could about my brain. My therapist, Lisa, encouraged me. She believed me, and that was what I needed the most. I had spent a lifetime being called a liar, though I tried so hard to be honest. After a lifetime of never being believed about even the most trivial things, finding someone who listened and believed me was somewhat uncomfortable. I had never had someone reassure me that I was not strange or broken beyond repair. Finding Lisa was an absolute gift.

As I delved deep into different topics of psychology, I discovered the covert narcissist, and my world exploded. I have never felt so seen. I have never felt so understood. These days narcissist is a well-known term, though not always used correctly. It was the covert part that really got me. The hidden narcissist. The one who chooses one scapegoat and shows the world an entirely false face of kindness and joy.

My family fits the mold perfectly, and I am the scapegoat. In the beginning, before I understood this whole dynamic, I called myself the family's emotional dumpster. It's essentially the same thing.

This was a major turning point. Being able to identify my issues and put a name to it has made it possible to heal. However refreshing it may have been to put a name to it, it certainly did not make healing any easier. Healing is inherently painful. Another lesson I have learned over the last couple of years is that if you want to heal from it, you have to feel it first.

Eventually, seeing the same painful patterns repeating over and over and watching it begin to affect my marriage and my kids, I had to take some major steps. I had to go no-contact with my mother.

This choice comes with a lot of stigma. The Mother Wound is very real, but people will still try to convince you that because she birthed you, she must love and respect you. Mine does not. I have confused manipulation with love all my life, and it has led me to some dark places. Places I never want to go again.

It felt like a veil had lifted from my eyes. I began to see things from a different perspective. Moments from my childhood, for which I had always assumed blame, became obviously twisted. A child is not capable of being at fault for some of the things I was holding blame for. Plus, who at 40 years old is still paying for the mistakes and misdeeds of their youth? Who is having that kind of stuff brought up numerous times a year?

Until therapy, I believed that this was normal, and it has twisted every relationship I have had in my adult life. The trauma was ongoing, and I was the only one who could stop it. My mother was not going to. Why would she?

Going no-contact has been the most difficult thing I have ever done, and the most beneficial. While the judgement has been severe, and I have lost my entire family except for my wonderful husband and kids, I have also found something I never thought I could have – self-respect. It seems like a very simple thing, but I have spent my entire life apologizing for taking up space, apologizing for being alive. I never felt deserving of the air I breathed. Now, I know that I deserve so much more.

I have also stopped binge eating. A lifetime of eating disorders and hating my body to the point of self-destruction, and when I finally made the choice to go no-contact, I stopped craving junk. I began to feel full. This moment was indescribable. I was confused at first and didn't understand what I was feeling, but when the realization came, I was filled with joy. My husband thought I was nuts when I got so excited to have normal full and hungry responses, but I had never felt them. I always felt empty. There was always a hole inside me, and it could never be filled.

When I was a kid, I was teased by my whole family for my voracious appetite. My grandmother said I had a "hollow leg." I was just never full. Now, I know it wasn't a hollow leg. It was a hollow heart, a need so deep and so painful that I had to eat to numb it. As a kid, it was my only option. As I got older, I tried everything I could think of to numb myself. I didn't want to feel because feeling was painful and meant that I needed to face the truth. It is incredibly hard to accept that your mother doesn't love you.

I know she just isn't capable. I know she had a rough life and is doing what she needs to do to cope, but I cannot help her. She doesn't want me to. She is comfortable where she is in life, and she would never be able to see things from my perspective. If allowed to continue, she would keep testing me, and I would keep failing.

Since going no-contact, she has tried every tactic in the book. She even tried to sow doubt into my perception of my mothering abilities. Luckily, I am beyond believing anything she says now, and I know in my heart that I am a good mother. My kids are happy, well-adjusted, and emotionally supported. I have always allowed them to be their own unique people, and I have always had their backs when life got difficult. I have no regrets in how I have raised them. It angers me that she would even try to make me doubt my choices, but I know it was a last-ditch effort to get me back under control. As for me, I've never been so solid in who I am and what I want. My newfound self-love and strength are intoxicating.

I wish the healing could have begun earlier. I often wonder what my life could have been like with emotional support, or if I had been allowed to go to therapy and get medications. What if I had been allowed to admit that I tried to end my life? It was kept quiet to save face for the family, and I was left to shove it deep down inside and agree to their chosen version of the story. That I was just trying to get attention. No one cared that

I wanted to die. No one questioned why a young girl would want to end a life that was just truly beginning. Instead, they created such a stigma in my mind about seeking help that I let myself drown for decades.

There is no going back, only forward. I am healing. Slowly, but I see the progress in my day-to-day activities. I am learning to set boundaries. I am learning how to handle the losses that some of these new boundaries cause. There have been quite a few. When you've been giving and giving and giving your whole life, people get upset when you take that away.

Still, with medication, therapy, and meditation I am calmer than I have ever been. I have learned what happiness feels like, and I am learning how to express my joy without fear of reprisal. I have a normal relationship with food and have actual hunger cues. I have found ways to love myself as I am at this moment. I finally value my own existence.

There is still a lot of anger, and it is going to take a long time to work through it all. Lisa told me recently that we are still at the beginning of our work. It shouldn't feel daunting since we've been working together for over two years already, but I know she's right. I had to climb out of the darkness and realize my worth before things could truly begin. I am excited for what is to come. I am 40 years old, and my life is just beginning.

There is one thing I can do about my messed-up past. One thing that is non-negotiable. It *has* to be done. I must stop the cycle. I have made a good start. I knew when my babies were born that there were a lot of things I wanted to do differently in raising them. Plus, an aching heart can also be overflowing with love that needs a place to go. My kids have benefited greatly from all that pent-up love.

Now, being raised by a covert narcissist causes all kinds of damage, and it tends to create narcissistic traits in everyone around them. The scapegoat is not immune. It has been incredibly uncomfortable facing these less than desirable traits in myself. It explains a lot about my actions in the past but confronting them still makes me cringe.

Still, the past is the past, and there is nothing to do to change it. By examining these actions and being honest with myself about my motivations and who I have been, I can heal myself and live a better, more authentic life moving forward.

I never planned on reaching 40. This part of my future was always hidden in shadow. I thought I would dread getting older, but now I know I'm just getting started.

If you are lost in the darkness, no matter how you ended up there, please know that you can get out. There is hope. It may only be the very slightest glint of light in an otherwise impenetrable dark, but it is there. You can find it, and when you do, hold onto it with everything you've got. Know that everything passes, and life can change in an instant. You may feel very lonely and isolated, but there are so many others going through the same type of thing. You are not alone. Find your people. It is not an easy task. I am still searching, but I have found a few of them. And, I have Lisa. I hope you can find your Lisa as well.

Just talk. Silence is the greatest oppressor. I suffered in silence for so long, holding onto everyone's secrets. Silence is heavy, and secrets are poison. Freedom comes with letting go. Tell your story. Reveal your truth. I never truly understood until now, but the truth *will* set you free. And what comes next is light.

Bio: Em Frappier is an author and podcast creator from the beautiful green mountains of Vermont. She is fascinated by the workings of the human mind and dedicated to understanding her own brain in the hopes of helping others.

MENTAL ILLNESS WITH A SLICE OF HUMBLE PIE

by Jessica Oakwood

"What are you grateful for?" I ask my friend.

We're sitting smoking on the step in the doorway of his Bristol flat, our legs dangling out onto the street. A bright mosaic of houses surrounds us.

He pulls up a fold out chair left there for this very purpose and assembles it like origami. My bare feet touch the concrete reassuringly.

"Shall I start at the beginning?" he asks. And he sits down deliberately, looking outwardly, as though the universe rests behind his eyes.

And so, he begins.

"I'm grateful that millions of years ago the planet formed, that it sustains life. I'm grateful that we evolved to exist. Humans. That we live and breathe and think. I'm grateful to be born, and grateful to live in a first world country. I'm grateful that I'm healthy. I'm grateful for my family and my friends. I'm grateful for the food I get every day. I'm grateful that I get to do what I love, and grateful that I had the luck and opportunities to let me get there. I'm grateful for this beautiful city, with its rich tapestry of diversity. I'm grateful for cute, cuddly things like puppies, which I think are adorable. I'm grateful for this moment, and grateful to be in it. I'm grateful that the world exists how it does today and I'm grateful for my small but meaningful place in it."

He says all this looking out of the doorway and watching the rings of smoke from our cigarettes float about in the air carelessly.

I notice a balloon flying overhead. Beetle green.

His eyes see more than just the paving stones around us. More than the bright eggshell blue front door a few meters away. More than the ethereal silver Fiat 500 someone has parked across the double yellow lines.

"What are you grateful for?" he asks.

"You," I say, trying not to cry.

***

Mental illness is humbling.

There's nothing like a persistent bout of psychosis to take you down a peg or two; to humble you; to make you feel grateful; to make you appreciate what you have and not what you don't have. I might not appreciate everything life has thrown at me, but I still strive to appreciate what I do have.

I appreciate the everyday now in a way that I don't think I did before. I appreciate kind actions and my friends with all the vivacity of someone about to drop dead at any moment. I appreciate bread fresh from the bakery and I appreciate the temperature of the floor beneath my feet. I appreciate that I am alive and breathing. Despite my newfound limitations in the world, I appreciate the morning and the afternoon and dusk. I appreciate first breakfast and second breakfast, too. I appreciate this essay and my fervor for typing and herding words around.

When people tell me to be grateful despite my illness, I feel like rolling my eyes. But there's something in that, despite my opposition. People with psychosis do not have good odds, 1 in 10 die by suicide – 30% are treatment resistant.

Amidst my unluckiness, I have become lucky. Grateful. Appreciative.

I appreciate the roof over my head and the health I do have even though the mental health I don't have seems to dominate and override everything else. I appreciate my friends and family who stuck by me through thick and thin. Literally – I've put on three stone compared to my angular limbs at crisis a few years ago. It's the antipsychotic meds, you see? I ate five pieces of toast every day in the mental health hospital, I was so hungry. Medicated hunger.

I appreciate the mental health care team who do their best to support me. I appreciate writing and talking about these experiences and the hope that it gives me.

They say sometimes you think you've been buried but you've actually been planted. And that's what I try to do – grow shoots from the dirt of rock bottom. Find hope even amidst all this chaos.

Life has dealt me a bad set of cards, but it doesn't mean the game is over. It just means I might have to play things a little different.

I appreciate being here in this moment and though I'd like to tweak my journey – erase the bits of my story I don't like., edit it to make it a happy ending – that's not a luxury I have unfortunately.

I appreciate this sheet of paper and the words on it. I appreciate who I have become BECAUSE of these experiences. Who they have made – me.

I appreciate fresh sheets and the smell after it rains.

I appreciate you.

Bio: Jessica Oakwood is a mental health writer and activist from Wiltshire, UK who has previously written for Mind, Rethink and Sane. She is autistic, sober, and suffers from schizoaffective disorder.

MENTAL HEALTH RESOURCES

ACTIVE MINDS

Active Minds is a nonprofit organization dedicated to promoting mental health, especially among young adults, via peer-to-peer dialogue and interaction. Active Minds was founded by Alison Malmon in 2003, after her older brother died by suicide in 2000. Learn more at *www.activeminds.org*.

ASIAN MENTAL HEALTH COLLECTIVE

It is the mission of AMHC to normalize and de-stigmatize mental health within the Asian community. AMHC aspires to make mental health easily available, approachable, and accessible to Asian communities worldwide. Learn more at *www.asianmhc.org*.

AMERICAN FOUNDATION FOR SUICIDE PREVENTION

The American Foundation for Suicide Prevention (AFSP) is a voluntary health organization that gives those affected by suicide a nationwide community empowered by research, education, and advocacy to take action against this leading cause of death. AFSP is dedicated to saving lives and bringing hope to those affected by suicide, including those who have experienced a loss. AFSP creates a culture that's smart about mental health by engaging in the following core strategies: Funding scientific research; Educating the public about mental health and suicide prevention; Advocating for public policies in mental health and suicide prevention; Supporting survivors of suicide loss and those affected by suicide. Learn more at *www.afsp.org*.

BLACK EMOTIONAL AND MENTAL HEALTH COLLECTIVE

BEAM is a training, movement building, and grant making institution that is dedicated to the healing, wellness, and liberation of Black and marginalized communities. Their mission is to remove the barriers that Black people experience getting access to or staying connected with emotional health care and healing through education, training, advocacy, and the creative arts. Learn more at *beam.community*.

INTERNATIONAL MENTAL HEALTH ASSOCIATION

IMHA began with a single project in Bangladesh and has grown into a global non-profit. Their mission is to build a healthier world through collaborative innovation. As a team, they work with communities around the world who are striving to bring change involving mental health. Currently, IMHA has team members based in Bangladesh, Canada, Kenya, Switzerland, and the United States. Their Advisors are based in Kenya, Nigeria, and Pakistan. IMHA currently partners with organizations from Bangladesh, Kenya, Uganda, the United States, and Zimbabwe. Learn more at *www.imha.ngo*.

MELANIN AND MENTAL HEALTH

Melanin & Mental Health® was born out of a desire to connect individuals with culturally competent clinicians committed to serving the mental health needs of Black and Latinx/Hispanic communities. They are committed to promoting the growth and healing of communities through our website, online directory, and monthly events. Learn more at *www.melaninandmentalhealth.com*.

NATIONAL ALLIANCE ON MENTAL ILLNESS

The National Alliance on Mental Illness (NAMI) is the largest grassroots mental health organization in the United States dedicated to building better lives for the millions of Americans affected by mental illness. NAMI provides advocacy, education, support and public awareness so that all individuals and families affected by mental illness can build better lives. Learn more at *www.nami.org*.

NATIONAL AMERICAN INDIAN AND ALASKA NATIVE MENTAL HEALTH TECHNOLOGY TRANSFER CENTER

The National American Indian and Alaska Native Mental Health Technology Transfer Center's mission is to ensure that American Indians and Alaska Natives have ready access to high-quality, evidence-based and experience-based, culturally appropriate, and self-directed behavioral health services and recovery supports – provided through a collaborative and integrative network of care – that effectively improves health and well-being. Learn more at *www.mhttcnetwork.org/centers/national-american-indian-and-alaska-native-mhttc/home*.

NATIONAL QUEER AND TRANS THERAPISTS OF COLOR NETWORK

The National Queer and Trans Therapists of Color Network (NQTTCN) is a healing justice organization committed to transforming mental health for queer and trans people of color (QTPoC). They work at the intersection of movements for social justice and the field of mental health to integrate healing justice into both of these spaces. Their overall goal is to increase access to healing justice resources for QTPoC. Learn more at *www.nqttcn.com*.

POETSIN

PoetsIN is The Creative Mental Health Charity created by Paul and Sammie, two individuals who have lived-experience of mental ill-health diagnoses stretching back to childhood and a shared experience of coping with their symptoms to keep them safe. It was this shared experience that motivated Paul and Sammie to utilize their creative coping and management strategies to give others a voice and help them on their journey to recovery and health. Learn more at *www.poetsin.com.*

PROJECT HEALTHY MINDS

Project Healthy Mins is a non-profit seeking to close the long-standing mental health treatment gap that has risen to catastrophic levels by fighting the continuing stigma around mental health and the difficulty in finding mental health treatment. They aim to build a free, consumer-friendly, one-stop digital referral platform that aims to increase access to care by making it fast and easy to find and navigate available resources. Learn more at *www.projecthealthyminds.com.*

THE TREVOR PROJECT

The Trevor Project is an American nonprofit organization founded in 1998. It focuses on suicide prevention efforts among lesbian, gay, bisexual, transgender, queer, and questioning youth. Through a toll-free telephone number, it operates The Trevor Lifeline, a confidential service that offers trained counselors. Learn more at *www.thetrevorproject.org.*

THIS IS MY BRAVE

This Is My Brave is a nonprofit organization that uses the performing arts to end stigma surrounding mental illness and addiction. Their mission is to empower individuals to put their names and faces on their true stories of recovery from mental illness and addiction. Since 2014, This Is My Brave has produced over 75 unique shows in cities across the United States featuring nearly 875 storytellers sharing true, personal stories on overcoming depression, anxiety, bipolar disorder, PTSD, psychosis, OCD, postpartum depression, borderline personality disorder, dissociative identity disorder, trichotillomania, anorexia, bulimia, sexual assault, alcoholism, substance use disorder and more. Learn more here *www.thisismybrave.org*.

WORLD HEALTH ORGANIZATION

The WHO has a division for mental health. It's a reliable source of information on mental health topics, including mental disorders. They provide facts and statistics worldwide and by region. They work worldwide and online to equip more than 7 billion people with better health, including mental health and wellbeing. WHO Mind engages in specific projects and creates policies to promote mental health services for everyone while providing helpful resources. Learn more at *www.who.int/teams/mental-health-and-substance-use.*

ACKNOWLEDGEMENTS

Putting together *Our Stories to Tell* has been a labor of love. Despite may setbacks and unforeseen issues, I was able to reach the finish line, but not without the help of some amazing individuals. I would like to thank Shenai Alonge-Moore for stepping in as copyeditor at the last minute, Will Dady of Renard Press for his incredible typesetting, and our Indiegogo supporters for their support and funding of the anthology. I also want to say a huge thank you to the contributors of this anthology for sticking with the project, even when the process seemed like it may never be complete. It takes a village to build something with great impact, and I'm so thankful for the village that built this anthology.

INDIEGOGO CONTRIBUTORS

Kaitlin Lopez
Alice Piotrowska
Amber Langehennig
Chellsey Tencati
Beth Lunney
Kenneth L Mahan
Natalie Stone
Denise Coger
Bob and Brenda Fields
Katie Kent
Deborah Todd
Christy Rogers
Amy Lee Guzman
Sunny Chen
Eve Brodsly
Elizabeth Woodward
Kimiko Vann
Seth Pritchett
David McDonald
Allie Carney
Ashley Orndorff
Carole Carroll
Trisha Martin
Shenai Alonge

Ange Harker
Kelly Witkins
Katie Baptist
Valerie Dimino
Sabrina Cargill-Greer
Stephanie Cargill-Greer
James W Johnson
Elizabeth Evans
Katelynn Young
Radhika Iyer
Maggie Ginsberg
Whitney Sheff
Heather Walder
Diana Beebe
Jess Witkins
Annlee Ellingson
Sarah Sooter
Taylor Guesnier
Kiersten Lipps

www.ingramcontent.com/pod-product-compliance
Lightning Source LLC
Chambersburg PA
CBHW072015210726
48294CB00011B/724
* 9 7 8 1 7 3 6 2 7 0 1 1 0 *